Substance Use Disorder - New Research Perspectives in the Diagnosis, Treatment, and Prognosis

Edited by Patricia Sampedro-Piquero, Román Darío Moreno Fernández and Clara Zancada-Menéndez

Published in London, United Kingdom

Substance Use Disorder - New Research Perspectives in the Diagnosis, Treatment, and Prognosis
http://dx.doi.org/10.5772/intechopen.100838
Edited by Patricia Sampedro-Piquero, Román Darío Moreno Fernández and Clara Zancada-Menéndez

Contributors
Gregory Rudolf, Zeng-Hui Ding, Yu-Xiang Qian, Cun-Feng Yuan, Xian-Jun Yang, Yu Liu, Yi-Ning Sun, Mu Wang, Sandeep Sitaram Kadu, Sayan Mondal, Anilendu Pramanik, Alojz Nociar, Stanislava Šaffová, Patricia Sampedro-Piquero, Román Darío Moreno Fernández, Clara Zancada-Menéndez

First published in London, United Kingdom, 2023 by IntechOpen
IntechOpen is the global imprint of INTECHOPEN LIMITED, registered in England and Wales, registration number: 11086078, 5 Princes Gate Court, London, SW7 2QJ, United Kingdom

British Library Cataloguing-in-Publication Data
A catalogue record for this book is available from the British Library

Additional hard and PDF copies can be obtained from orders@intechopen.com

Substance Use Disorder - New Research Perspectives in the Diagnosis, Treatment, and Prognosis
Edited by Patricia Sampedro-Piquero, Román Darío Moreno Fernández and Clara Zancada-Menéndez
p. cm.
Print ISBN 978-1-80356-275-9
Online ISBN 978-1-80356-276-6
eBook (PDF) ISBN 978-1-80356-277-3

Meet the editors

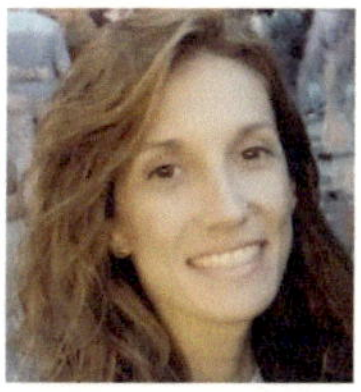

Patricia Sampedro-Piquero is an assistant professor in the Faculty of Psychology, at the Autonomous University of Madrid. She has developed a line of research focused on cognitive and/or emotional alterations linked to fields such as aging and substance use, as well as the role of non-pharmacological interventions in their treatment. In addition, she has been the principal investigator of two projects related to cognitive deficits and substance use and is currently part of the research team of two projects focused on neurophysiological alterations related to heavy alcohol consumption in adolescents and the role of neuropsychology in the assessment and treatment of addiction. She has several journal articles and book chapters to her credit.

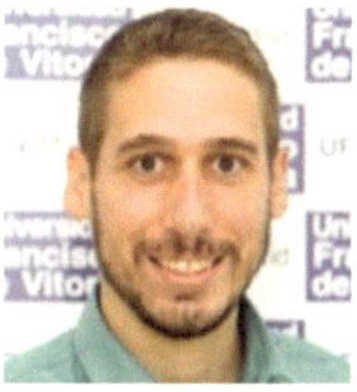

Roman Moreno Fernandez has a Ph.D. in Psychology from the University of Malaga, Spain. He has published thirteen articles in high-impact scientific journals such as Translational Psychiatry of Nature and Disease Models & Mechanisms. He has completed two international stays at the Brain Mind Institute (BMI), in Switzerland, and a national short stay at Instituto Cajal (CSIC). He has one patent and more than twenty communications in international congresses to his credit.

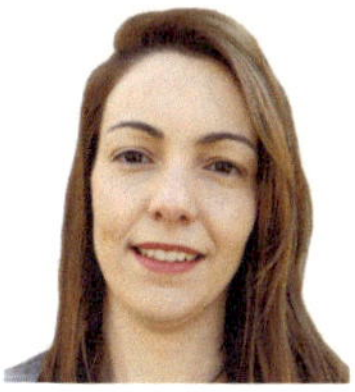

Clara Zancada Menendez is a specialist in neuropsychology with a Ph.D. in Psychology from the University of Oviedo, Spain. She has carried out numerous research stays at universities including Harvard University, USA and Vanderbilt University, USA. Her research involves using new technologies such as immersive virtual reality environments to study the influence of aging on cognitive processes. She has also conducted research in animal models to ascertain the influence of factors such as cognitive reserve, enrichment, and exercise on the brain during aging processes.

Contents

Preface

Adolescence is a particularly vulnerable period of neurodevelop¬ment in which the incorrect management of emotional, social, and behavioral changes can lead to unsuccessful adulthood. During this period of life the brain is still maturing, being a moment of dynamic specialization of core brain systems, particularly the frontal structures. Earlier initiation of substance use in adolescence is associated not only with an increased risk of dependence but also with antisocial behavior and impairments of adaptive functioning, including relationship difficulties, academic failure, unemployment, and mental health issues. This book presents a comprehensive overview of multidisciplinary issues about adolescence and substance abuse, with a special focus on alcohol. Written by experts in the field, chapters discuss risk factors related to the onset and maintenance of substance abuse in adolescence, behavioral and pharmacological approaches to prevent and/or reduce the negative consequences of substance abuse, and psychological disorders associated with drug abuse.

Dr. Patricia Sampedro-Piquero,
Faculty of Psychology,
Autonomous University of Madrid,
Madrid, Spain

Dr. Román Darío Moreno Fernández
Faculty of Psychology,
Universidad Francisco de Vitoria,
Madrid, Spain

Dr. Clara Zancada-Menéndez
Faculty of Psychology,
The International University of La Rioja,
Logroño, Spain

Section 1

Introduction

Chapter 1

Introductory Chapter: Adolescent Substance Abuse – Risk Factors and Consequences

Patricia Sampedro-Piquero, Clara Zancada-Menéndez and Román Darío Moreno Fernández

1. Introduction

1.1 Adolescence and substance abuse

People are most likely to begin abusing drugs (including tobacco, cannabis, alcohol, and other illicit substances) during adolescence and young adulthood from ages 10 to 19 [1]. Adolescence is a particularly vulnerable period of neurodevelopment in which the incorrect management of emotional, social, and behavioral changes can lead to an unsuccessful adulthood [2]. Regarding the brain anatomy and function, it is well known that during this period of life the brain is still maturating, being a moment of dynamic specialization of core brain systems, particularly the frontal structures [3]. In fact, the neural plasticity that occurs during this period creates a unique opportunity to influence the behavioral and developmental trajectories [4]. It is also a difficult period in which a high percentage of their decisions rely more on an emotional response or even on the social rewards rather than in a logical response. Therefore, as Hall noted in 1904, adolescence is a period of *storm and stress* (revised in [5]) because adolescents are characterized by a greater impulsivity, and less control over impulses, behaviors, and emotions, as well as a heightened reward sensitivity [6, 7]. As consequence, these personality, cognitive and behavioral patterns contribute to the emergence of risky and disruptive behaviors, such as drug abuse, which is common in Western countries [8].

This increased propensity to consume drugs is also enhanced by the fact that adolescents tend to be significantly less sensitive to their effects than adults [9]. Hence, adolescents experience less hangover symptoms and negative affect during alcohol withdrawal [10]. Besides, longitudinal studies have also suggested that impulsivity and the lack of inhibitory control could predict early onset drinking and alcohol dependence [11, 12]. On the other hand, alcohol consumption can promote itself impulsive actions by impairing basic inhibitory process [13]. Specifically, adolescents often consumed alcohol in repeated short episodes of heavy intake followed by detoxification and extended periods of abstinence, known as binge drinking (BD) [14]. This drinking pattern consists in drinking 5 or more glasses of alcoholic beverages in short periods of time (2 h) increasing the blood alcohol concentration above 80 mg/dl [15, 16]. Several preclinical and clinical studies have revealed that BD is associated with long-term behavioral and neurobiological impairments along with a risk of dependence in adulthood [17]. Nowadays, it is estimated that 40% of people between the ages of 15 and 24 engage in this pattern of alcohol consumption, which contributes to several medical complications, as well as higher risk of developing alcohol use disorder [18]. Further, the potential role of substance use as a risk factor for adult psychiatric disorders and dependence is remarkable [19]. These negative consequences are due in part to the drugs impact on brain mechanisms and signaling systems, whose maturation mainly happens during adolescence [9]. Thereby, in general, early drug exposure can produce impairments in the brain structure and function, resulting in several emotional, behavioral, and cognitive deficits [20]. For instance, studies have revealed persistent alcohol-induced neurobiological changes within the prefrontal cortex, the hippocampus, and the amygdala integrally involved in governing diverse emotional states [21–23].

Earlier initiation of substance use in adolescence is associated not only with an increased risk of dependence but also with antisocial behavior and impairments of adaptive functioning, including relationship difficulties, academic failure, unemployment, and mental health issues [24–26]. Besides, over half of the adolescents receiving treatment will relapse within 1 year of treatment [27], suggesting more accessible and effective programs needed to prevent and treat substance abuse in adolescents. Consequently, there is a need to explore other alternatives to treatment that, alone or in combination with existing ones, representing an improvement in treatment [28, 29].

Despite the relevance and clear influence of personality and neuropsychological factors in the development of substance abuse behaviors, we should not neglect the study of the impact of family dynamics and the social environment in which these young people live as possible predisposing variables. Regarding family factors, some studies have observed that young people who engage in substance abuse perceive a lower quality of family functioning with lower levels of cohesion, flexibility, communication, satisfaction, and a higher degree of disengagement compared with healthy adolescents [30]. Moreover, living in families that are not very flexible, highly disengaged and with communication problems among their members, is also a risk factor, suggesting the importance of prevention programs being based on an integrated approach focused also on improving the family environment. On the other hand, it has been observed that children of parents who also have addiction problems are more likely to present excessive consumption of drugs [31]. Nevertheless, there is also literature that did not find a significant association between parental drug consumption and substance abuse in adolescence [32]. Finally, another important social factor, especially for young people, is their use of social networks. Thus, it has been observed that the content of these is poorly regulated, tending to use marketing tactics based on the vulnerability of young people to the image, social relationships, and their need to fit in with the group [33]. To date, there is little work that has investigated the behavioral profiles of young people with drug-related problems on social networks, although this could have interesting implications for treatment and prevention. **Figure 1** summarizes different risk factors involved in substance abuse during adolescence.

Therefore, this book presents a comprehensive overview of multidisciplinary issues about adolescence and substance abuse, especially focus on alcohol. It has been written to be consulted by students and professionals of multiple psychological, biological, and social disciplines. Chapters has been also written for academics and researchers on different areas focusing on risk factors related to the onset and

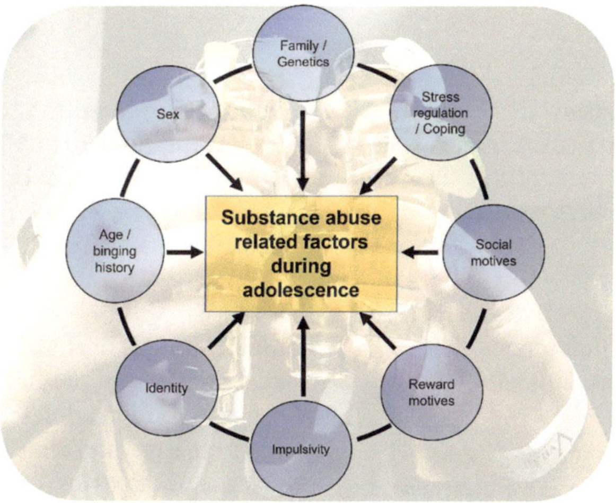

Figure 1.
Variables associated with drug abuse during the adolescence and youth.

maintenance of substance abuse in adolescence, as well as potential of behavioral and pharmacological approaches to prevent and/or reduced the negative consequences involved in substance abuse. Finally, psychological disorders associated with drug abuse are also considered in this book.

Author details

Patricia Sampedro-Piquero[1]*, Clara Zancada-Menéndez[2] and Román Darío Moreno Fernández[3]

1 Facultad de Psicología, Departamento de Psicología Biológica y de la Salud, Universidad Autónoma de Madrid, Spain

2 Facultad de Psicología, Universidad Internacional de la Rioja (UNIR), Spain

3 Facultad de Educación y Psicología, Universidad Francisco de Vitoria, Spain

*Address all correspondence to: patricia.sampedro@uam.es

References

[1] Nawi AM, Ismail R, Ibrahim F, Hassan MR, Manaf MRA, Amit N, et al. Risk and protective factors of drug abuse among adolescents: A systematic review. BMC Public Health. 2021;**21**:2088

[2] Steinberg L. Cognitive and affective development in adolescence. Trends in Cognitive Sciences. 2005;**9**:69-74

[3] Vijayakumar N, Op de Macks Z, Shirtcliff EA, Pfeifer JH. Puberty and the human brain: Insights into adolescent development. Neuroscience and Biobehavioral Reviews. 2018;**92**:417-436

[4] Spear LP. The adolescent brain and age-related behavioral manifestations. Neuroscience and Biobehavioral Reviews. 2000;**24**:417-463

[5] Arnett JJ. Adolescent storm and stress, reconsidered. American Psychologist. 1999;**54**:317-326

[6] Casey BJ. Beyond simple models of self-control to circuit-based accounts of adolescent behavior. Annual Review of Psychology. 2015;**66**:295-319

[7] Rømer D, Reyna VF, Satterthwaite TD. Beyond stereotypes of adolescent risk taking: Placing the adolescent brain in developmental context. Developmental Cognitive Neuroscience. 2017;**27**:19-34

[8] Degenhardt L, Stockings E, Patton G, Hall WD, Lynskey M. The increasing global health priority of substance use in young people. The Lancet Psychiatry. 2016;**3**:251-264

[9] Spear LP. Effects of adolescent alcohol consumption on the brain and behaviour. Nature Reviews. Neuroscience. 2018;**19**:197-214

[10] Lees B, Meredith LR, Kirkland AE, Bryant BE, Squeglia LM. Effect of alcohol use on the adolescent brain and behavior. Pharmacology, Biochemistry, and Behavior. 2020;**192**:172906

[11] Ernst M, Luckenbaugh DA, Moolchan ET, Leff MK, Allen R, Eshel N, et al. Behavioral predictors of substance-use initiation in adolescents with and without attention-deficit/hyperactivity disorder. Pediatrics. 2006;**117**:2030-2039

[12] Rømer Thomsen K, Callesen MB, Hesse M, Kvamme TL, Pedersen MM, Pedersen MU, et al. Impulsivity traits and addiction-related behaviors in youth. Journal of Behavioral Addictions. 2018;**7**:317-330

[13] de Wit H. Impulsivity as a determinant and consequence of drug use: A review of underlying processes. Addiction Biology. 2009;**14**:22-31

[14] Chung T, Creswell KG, Bachrach R, Clark DB, Martin CS. Adolescent binge drinking. Alcohol Research. 2018;**39**:5-15

[15] Alessandrini G, Ciccarelli R, Battagliese G, Lombardo G, De Rosa F, Messina MP, et al. Interdisciplinary Study Group CRARL - SITAC - SIPaD - SITD - SIPDip. Treatment of alcohol dependence. Alcohol and the young: Social point of view. Rivista di Psichiatria. 2018;**53**:113-117

[16] Gunzerath L, Faden V, Zakhari S, Warren K. National Institute on Alcohol Abuse and Alcoholism report on moderate drinking. Alcoholism, Clinical and Experimental Research. 2004;**28**:829-847

[17] Jones SA, Lueras JM, Nagel BJ. Effects of binge drinking on the developing

brain. Alcohol Research: Current Reviews. 2018;**39**:87-96

[18] Lannoy S, Billieux J, Dormal V, Maurage P. Behavioral and cerebral impairments associated with binge drinking in youth: A critical review. Psychologica Belgica. 2019;**59**:116-155

[19] Stoddard SA, Eisman A, Aiyer S, Zimmerman MA. The transition from adolescence to adulthood and associated substance use/abuse. Adolescent Medicine: State of the Art Reviews. 2013;**24**:611-620

[20] El Marroun H, Klapwijk ET, Koevoets M, Brouwer RM, Peters S, Van't Ent D, et al. Alcohol use and brain morphology in adolescence: A longitudinal study in three different cohorts. The European Journal of Neuroscience. 2021;**54**:6012-6026

[21] Jadhav KS, Boutrel B. Prefrontal cortex development and emergence of self-regulatory competence: The two cardinal features of adolescence disrupted in context of alcohol abuse. The European Journal of Neuroscience. 2019;**50**:2274-2281

[22] Sakharkar AJ, Kyzar EJ, Gavin DP, Zhang H, Chen Y, Krishnan HR, et al. Altered amygdala DNA methylation mechanisms after adolescent alcohol exposure contribute to adult anxiety and alcohol drinking. Neuropharmacology. 2019;**157**:107679

[23] Walker CD, Kuhn CM, Risher ML. The effects of peri-adolescent alcohol use on the developing hippocampus. International Review of Neurobiology. 2021;**160**:251-280

[24] Behrendt S, Wittchen HU, Höfler M, Lieb R, Beesdo K. Transitions from first substance use to substance use disorders in adolescence: Is early onset associated with a rapid escalation? Drug and Alcohol Dependence. 2009;**99**:68-78

[25] Guttmannova K, Hill KG, Bailey JA, Lee JO, Hartigan LA, Hawkins JD, et al. Examining explanatory mechanisms of the effects of early alcohol use on young adult alcohol dependence. Journal of Studies on Alcohol and Drugs. 2012;**73**:379-390

[26] Slade T, Chapman C, Swift W, Keyes K, Tonks Z, Teesson M. Birth cohort trends in the global epidemiology of alcohol use and alcohol-related harms in men and women: Systematic review and metaregression. BMJ Open. 2016;**6**:e011827

[27] Ramo DE, Brown SA. Classes of substance abuse relapse situations: A comparison of adolescents and adults. Psychology of Addictive Behaviors. 2008;**22**:372-379

[28] Macht V, Crews FT, Vetreno RP. Neuroimmune and epigenetic mechanisms underlying persistent loss of hippocampal neurogenesis following adolescent intermittent ethanol exposure. Current Opinion in Pharmacology. 2020;**50**:9-16

[29] Sampedro-Piquero P, Moreno-Fernandez RD, Begega A, López M, Santín LJ. Consequences of alcohol use in early adolescence on emotional and cognitive status of mice in the late adolescence and adulthood: Focus on neuroadaptations in GR, CRF and BDNF. Addiction Biology. 2022;**27**:e13158

[30] Laghi F, Bianchi D, Pompili S, Lonigro A, Baiocco R. Binge eating and binge drinking behaviors: The role of family functioning. Psychology, Health & Medicine. 2021;**26**:408-420

[31] Skala K, Walter H. Adolescence and alcohol: A review of the literature. Neuropsychiatry. 2013;**27**:202-211

[32] Cable N, Sacker A. Typologies of alcohol consumption in adolescence: Predictors and adult outcomes. Alcohol and Alcoholism. 2008;**43**:81A90

[33] Rounsefell K, Gibson S, McLean S, Blair M, Molenaar A, Brennan L, et al. Social media, body image and food choices in healthy young adults: A mixed methods systematic review. Nutrition Diet. 2020;**77**:19-40

Section 2

New Researches

Chapter 2

Management of Co-Occurring SUD and Chronic Pain

Gregory Rudolf

Abstract

Though there has been a 44.4% decrease in the number of prescriptions written for opioid analgesics between the years 2011–2020 in the United States, drug overdose rates continue to climb sharply, reaching nearly 107,000 for a prior 12-months period as of early 2022, driven primarily by the use of illicit opioids. It is estimated that 80–90% of individuals with a substance use disorder (SUD) receive no treatment, and for those with opioid use disorder (OUD) who do find their way to treatment, less than half are offered potentially life-saving medication. Contemporaneously, chronic pain is one of the most common and most disabling health conditions, and frequently involves complex decision-making between the patient and the health care team regarding the treatment approach. Though prescribing trends have ebbed in recent years, opioids continue to be the most prescribed class of drug in the United States despite well-publicized associated harms. It is more critical than ever that stakeholders urgently work to facilitate and destigmatize evidence-based substance use disorder treatment, and promote safe, effective, and holistic care pathways for patients suffering from chronic pain.

Keywords: chronic pain, opioid use disorder, prescription opioids, substance use

1. Introduction

The "opioid crisis" as a major public health problem in the United States has been prominently recognized in medical literature and the press for at least a decade. Prompted by a variety of factors, the first of three defined "waves" of the crisis began with a dramatic increase in written prescriptions for opioid analgesics starting in the mid-1990's [1]. In lockstep with the surge in opioid prescribing, there was a coincident fourfold increase in overdose deaths and admissions to substance use disorder treatment programs. In 2015, more than 33,000 Americans died of opioid overdoses, and an estimated 2 million individuals suffered from substance use disorders related to prescription opioids [2].

There were multiple factors contributing to a threefold increase in the number of opioid prescriptions written in the United States between 1999 and 2011 [3]. The first relates to changing clinical practice norms, where indications for use of opioids for the treatment of chronic non-cancer pain widened significantly in response to escalating concerns about perceived widespread undertreatment of chronic pain. For example, at that time, the American Pain Society in its 1996 guidelines encouraged providers to assess pain as "the fifth vital sign" at each clinical encounter to avoid failing to actively address patients' pain symptoms. At the same time, aggressive marketing of opioids by pharmaceutical manufacturers, particularly the makers of Oxycontin™ following its 1996 FDA approval, served to amplify and drive this shift in prescribing culture, with sophisticated methodologies to increase provider prescribing patterns, and with the dissemination of now-discredited scientific information alleging low risk of misuse or addiction related to prescription opioids [4]. Payers limited access to other evidence-based pain interventions such as multidisciplinary pain rehabilitation, bodywork treatment, and psychological counseling, and these modalities of treatment thus became more difficult to access, increasing patients' reliance on pharmacotherapy, and doctors' willingness to prescribe opioids. Taken together, these factors created a prescribing climate which normalized opioids as a common treatment for chronic non-cancer pain [3].

Alongside the challenge of containing the harms caused by overprescription of opioid analgesics exists the very high prevalence and burden of suffering from chronic pain. The debilitating effects of chronic pain on quality of life involve not only physical symptoms, but also emotional well-being, identity, and interpersonal relationships [3]. Among patients with chronic pain who are newly prescribed opioids for longer than 90 days, approximately 6% develop OUD, with the likelihood increasing dramatically with an escalation in dose and extended duration [5]. In 2016, the Centers for Disease Control and Prevention issued guidelines for prescribing opioids for chronic pain which recommended soft limitations on dose levels to lower than 90 mg morphine equivalents per day (MED), and implementation of clinical practices to assess and prevent harm to use and misuse, such as urine toxicology screening and use of state prescription monitoring program [6]. This document strongly influenced prescriber practices nationwide, contributing to a general decrease of 40–60% in aggregate opioid prescriptions across the US from peak levels in the mid-2000s. Unfortunately, not all consequences of this shift in prescribing patterns have been positive. Many patients who had been using opioids over the long term, especially at higher doses, were forced by their prescriber to undergo dose tapering or discontinuation despite evident clinical stability, due to misapplication of the CDC guidelines, with associated harmful adverse events and outcomes, including increased rates of illicit drug use, emergency department visits and hospitalizations, and overdose deaths [7]. There have been recent attempts to better understand the disruptive power these changing norms and policies have continued to have on patients' pain management experiences [8].

This change in prescribing practices and the resultant barrier to patients receiving prescription opioids legitimately for pain was exacerbated by abrupt closures of "pill mill" clinics by law enforcement. These clinics operated on a profit-based model and provided substandard care and monitoring while prescribing outsized quantities of opioids and other controlled substances. As a result of these factors, proactive networks of drug traffickers primarily from Mexico were able to capitalize on a ready-made source of demand for cheaper and more reliably available illicit opioids, ushering in the second wave of the opioid crisis by 2015: increased heroin use [1, 9]. Sources from Mexico accounted for 90% of the US heroin market share by 2016 [9, 10]. Within a few more years, fentanyl, a synthetic opioid that is much cheaper, more potent, and easier to manufacture and distribute than heroin, took over the illicit opioid market. Showing no signs of slowing, fentanyl-related overdose death rates have only worsened as the so-called third wave of the opioid crisis continues [1].

In this context, management of chronic pain in the US has undergone systematic re-examination to elucidate best practices for patient safety and treatment effectiveness [8]. Elsewhere in the world, countries are attempting to learn from the mistakes of the US and prevent or mitigate major prescription opioid-related public health problems [11]. As providers are regularly tasked to straddle the intersecting realms of chronic pain disorders, substance use and mental health disorders, treatment approaches must emphasize evidence-based, compassionate, inclusive, patient-centered, safe, and sustainable interventions. Effective solutions to the crisis will include not only optimization of care delivery, but also relevant non-clinical aspects such as the roles of law enforcement and drug marketing and regulation [12]. Some countries have already made a marked shift in policy toward harm reduction, such as Canada, which has provided safe consumption sites for drug users, and the Netherlands and Portugal, which have decriminalized all drug use in favor of approaches emphasizing safety and access to treatment [13]. Though these measures have improved opioid-related death rates, countries outside the US have seen use of prescription opioids grow substantially (47% increase in Europe between 2004 and 2016) even though it is illegal to market drugs directly to patients in Europe and other parts of the world [13].

In this chapter, we will review the complex intersection of SUD and chronic pain disorders in several subcategories: 1) understanding the scope of the problem and its neurobiological underpinnings, including risk factors, and biopsychosocial mechanisms of chronic pain and substance use disorders; 2) the controversial role of opioids in chronic pain care; 3) best practices in chronic pain and SUD treatment.

2. Key concepts in understanding Co-occurring chronic pain and SUD

2.1 Epidemiology and neurobiology

The prevalence of either regional or widespread chronic pain in adults has been estimated at 30% [14]. About 20% of US adults (50 million people) report a moderate to severe level of pain which affects their daily quality of life and activity, while in the United Kingdom, chronic pain is estimated to affect 20–50% of the adult population. Worldwide, chronic low back pain is the single leading cause of disability across all age ranges, genders, and demographics [15]. Several other chronic pain conditions including chronic headache and peripheral joint pain from arthritis are also in the top 10 causes of disability worldwide. Factors that are consistently associated with disability from chronic low back pain include older age, poor general health, increased psychological or psychosocial stress, worse baseline functional disability, sciatica, and the presence of compensation related to disability [5]. Social determinants of health that are known to predict poor outcomes related to disability from chronic low back pain include low socioeconomic status and/or low income, unemployment, and occupational factors such as lack of adequate support staff, manual lifting, and frequent overtime work hours [16].

The prevalence of opioid use disorder (OUD) in patients with chronic pain has been notoriously difficult to determine with specificity. Through the historical lens of the opioid crisis, it was dramatically underestimated in the years preceding and including the spike in opioid prescribing starting in the 1990s. In a letter that was published in 1980 in the New England Journal of Medicine, authors Porter and Jick described a crude study in which charts were pulled for patients in a hospitalized setting who had been given opioids for a variety of indications, with neither dosing nor duration of treatment identified. The investigators concluded that only 4 of these 11,882 hospitalized patients that were treated with an opioid medication were subsequently diagnosed with an "addiction". Unfortunately, this study was widely cited as "proof" that there was only about a 1% risk that a patient treated with opioids for pain (even in an outpatient setting, even long-term) would develop opioid addiction. More recently, it has been recognized that the real prevalence of OUD is much higher, with various estimates ranging from 3.2 to 27%, with most of these estimates falling in the 20–25% range [17]. Though the level of prescription opioid use, and opioid-related deaths in most European countries and worldwide is still much lower than that of the US, as noted above Europe has seen a steady increase in prescription opioid use over the past 15 years, mainly due to increased tramadol, fentanyl, and oxycodone prescriptions; there are calls for proactive investigation into these trends and their potential subsequent harms [11].

Over the past several decades, significant progress has been made in understanding the neurobiology of pain and addiction. CNS receptor binding targets and associated neural circuitry has been elucidated to explain the rewarding effects of substances with known abuse potential. Moreover, we know that repeated drug exposure over time causes adaptations in the brain's reward pathways which are evident even on a gross structural level via neuroimaging [17]. Affected areas include the following:

- *the limbic system*: contains the brain's reward circuitry, leading to a drive to repeat behaviors that activate this pathway, such as using drugs

- *the brain stem*: controls basic functions critical to life such as heart rate and breathing

- *the cerebral cortex*: controls functioning via multiple sub-regions that govern thinking, feeling, sensory experience, motor coordination, planning, and decision-making.

Substances with potential for abuse that affect these areas of the brain, such as alcohol, opioids, cannabis, stimulants, sedatives, and nicotine, enhance specific brain neurochemical pathways in ways similar to that produced by other natural rewards such as food and sex, but in a sometimes more acutely intense and prolonged manner. Conversely, when long-term use of such substance is interrupted, a pronounced sense of dysphoria is typically experienced, which has been referred to as *hyperkatifeia* [18]. The threat of this unpleasant state produces a desire to avoid interruption in use, due to the behavioral negative reinforcement that the undesired state exerts over the individual, who otherwise recognizes the benefits of stopping the behavior and genuinely prefers and seeks to do so. In addition, the rewarding effect of use is itself diminished with prolonged use as tolerance is developed to the effects of the substance, and the ability of natural rewards to activate the reward pathways is likewise compromised. In this fashion, over time, these substances strongly influence the choices and behavior of the individual [19].

Chronic pain is best viewed as a distinct diagnosis and medical condition, with its own definition and taxonomy [14]. It has been associated with multiple physical, psychological, and social factors which affect its level of impact on a given individual [15]. The diagnosis of a chronic pain disorder can be made based on objective evaluation, as with an imaging test or a blood test, for example, with relatively clear etiology and a specifically identifiable pain generator. However, even in cases where the diagnosis is clear, patients with very similar objective findings might have a completely different "pain experience" based on other less quantifiable factors. These include:

- their level of central nervous system-mediated pain sensitivity or pain tolerance, which itself may be influenced by both genetic and environmental factors;
- their current psycho-emotional state and prior mental health history;
- the effect of the medications or substances they are using on pain processing pathways;
- other factors which can influence pain signaling and processing in the central nervous system (CNS) such as the history of trauma or adverse childhood experience (ACE), and attitudes/beliefs about pain [6].

Moreover, many chronic pain disorders are not typically associated with specific identifiable anatomic pathology. In the case of chronic low back pain, 85–95% of patients presenting to primary care providers do not have a clearly identifiable etiology for their symptoms [5]. Some pain syndromes are inherently caused or defined by a CNS-mediated pain state, such as fibromyalgia (prevalence estimated at 2–8% of the population). Other examples of this include headache syndromes, irritable bowel syndrome, temporomandibular joint syndrome, and interstitial cystitis. It should be noted, however, that what may have started as a focal, well-defined pain condition, such as low back pain from degenerative disc disease or lumbar facet arthropathy, may become a chronic, CNS-mediated pain state, such as in the case of failed surgical back syndrome [20]. Thus, it is incumbent upon care providers to recognize the complex role of the CNS in all chronic pain states, and to utilize treatment approaches that address the patient as a whole person rather than just as a structural or anatomic abnormality [21].

Pain can generally be subdivided into three general types, including nociceptive, inflammatory, and neuropathic [12]. Nociceptive pain is our bodies' sensory response to an actual painful stimulus, divided further into visceral (such as gastrointestinal) and somatic (such as musculoskeletal) pain. Inflammatory pain is a biological response within the body to facilitate tissue repair due to injury and can be either acute or chronic in nature. Acute inflammatory pain is exemplified by a sprained ankle, whereas chronic inflammatory pain is exemplified by osteoarthritis of a peripheral joint such as the hip. Neuropathic pain is typically defined by nerve injury or impairment leading to central pain sensitization (defined below), which results in a persistent pain response without a stimulus and is generally pathologic or maladaptive because it does not serve a useful purpose. Both the CNS and the peripheral nervous system (PNS) are involved in all 3 types of pain. The PNS comprises nerves and ganglia outside the brain and spinal cord, which define the CNS.

An individual's response to pain signals can be viewed in a general sense as either adaptive or maladaptive, with their emotional state playing a key role in this determination. In a person with normal pain sensitivity, pain signals from a twisting back injury would be transmitted from the dorsal horn of the spinal cord through ascending spinal pathways to be received by the brain, and the signals would then be modulated by descending inhibitory interneuron signals which serve to dampen the severity of the excitatory pain signals, in accordance with the now-classic gate control theory of pain as first proposed by Melzack and Wall in 1965, still supported in concept by the International Association for the Study of Pain [5]. Facilitating less distress and greater functional capacity, this normal sequence of pain processing is considered adaptive to the organism and species.

The same pain stimulus could be processed quite differently for a patient with chronic pain. Due to the emotional response caused by chronic pain signals, the inhibitory interneuron modulation of the descending pathway could be decreased, which leads to an increase in relative excitatory pain signaling input, with some relief coming from accompanying increase in endorphin release from the periaqueductal gray (PAG) and the dorsal horn of the spinal cord. Over time, via a process termed central sensitization, pain processing in the CNS recalibrates to adjusted thresholds for modulation of both ascending excitatory and descending inhibitory signals, resulting in the patient experiencing greater baseline pain sensitivity, and a higher level of distress with exacerbations of pain. The affective or emotional component, then, is recognized to have a significant influence on the ongoing physical experience of pain [22]. Moreover, this increased baseline pain sensitivity does not serve a functional purpose and would therefore be considered maladaptive [5].

When exogenous opioids are added longitudinally to this scenario, there is an accompanying decrease in the production and release of pain-relieving endogenous opioids from the PAG and dorsal horn, resulting in an increase in pain signaling along the ascending pathway. In addition to these effects on pain processing, prolonged opioids will also affect the pain experience by influencing the brain's limbic system (emotional circuitry, see below) and sleep patterns. These gradual changes in the CNS persist, even long after the opioid has been discontinued [19]. Such long-term CNS changes clearly have major implications in designing and implementing effective treatment approaches for both chronic pain and opioid use disorder/opioid physiologic dependence.

Despite the gains in knowledge and active investigation into the neurophysiology of pain and addiction, there is still a great deal that is incompletely understood. Much of our knowledge comes from laboratory and animal studies rather than from the actual patients who present for care. The influence of environmental factors such as trauma, for example, has been studied and shown to be quite impactful on the development of pain sensitivity, cognitive capability, memory, emotional resilience, and the likelihood of developing a SUD [17]. Also, very influential is the role of organic mental illness on the behaviors and brain function of a patient with chronic pain. In addition, issues such as genetics, social/housing instability, discriminatory disparities in accessing health care, and others, are known to greatly affect clinical outcomes for all patients experiencing chronic pain and addiction [6].

2.2 The duality of opioids: a brief review of general opioid pharmacology

Opioids have played a central role in the relief of human suffering for millennia; they are also a direct cause of great harm. They are a class of prescription drugs derived from the opium poppy plant, some directly and some via laboratory synthesis using similar chemical structures. They contain chemicals that can relieve pain and relax the body. They can also produce a euphoric effect which gives them potential for misuse. Further, they can induce depression of the respiratory drive, leading to an overdose death. For these reasons, prescription opioids are regulated by the Drug Enforcement Agency of the US government, and by analogous agencies elsewhere. Some common examples of prescription opioids are oxycodone, morphine, hydrocodone, codeine, tramadol, fentanyl, buprenorphine, and methadone. In individuals with co-occurring chronic pain and SUD, consideration of treatment with the use of opioids or other controlled substances that have the potential to be misused and cause harm is a common clinical dilemma for health care providers, as well as a quality assurance and risk management issue for policymakers. In the years since the advent of the current opioid crisis, which as noted above began with exponential increases in the widespread use of prescription opioids to treat chronic non-cancer pain, there has been increased effort to define best practices for dispensing prescription opioids for appropriate indications, for appropriate patients, and for the appropriate length of time [23].

Opioids can be classified in various ways, such as by potency, half-life, opioid receptor activity, or specific opioid chemical class. It is useful to start with categorizing opioids based on the way they are synthesized:

- *endogenous opioids*: opioid peptides produced organically by the body itself; examples are endorphins, enkephalins, dynorphins.

- *exogenous non-synthetic opioid agonists*: opioids derived from the opium poppy plant; examples are codeine, morphine, thebaine, diacetylmorphine (heroin).

- *exogenous semi-synthetic opioid agonists*: opioids derived from the poppy plant that have been chemically altered in the laboratory; examples are oxycodone, hydrocodone, hydromorphone.

- *exogenous synthetic opioid agonists*: opioids that are synthesized entirely in a laboratory; examples are methadone, fentanyl, buprenorphine.

Opioid pharmacodynamics, or the activity of the drug at the opioid receptor and the resultant physiologic and clinically relevant response, is at the heart of the question of how these drugs can be safely and effectively administered by clinicians [24]. Potency is certainly a key factor in this equation, and it is important that medical providers have a solid understanding of the relative potencies and basic pharmacologic properties of various opioid medications. Ranging from opioid partial agonists such as tramadol to high potency full agonists such as fentanyl, these potencies are classified by the World Health Organization on their "Analgesic Ladder" [11]. Of note, opioids with the highest potency also have the greatest addiction liability and highest risk of overdose death. The recent emergence of illicit synthetic analogs of fentanyl on the street has exposed users to levels of potency not seen before in clinical medicine; carfentanil, one such analog, is 100 times more potent than prescription fentanyl, which is itself 100 times more potent than morphine [25]. It is therefore not surprising that even users who are very experienced with other less potent opioids are highly susceptible to overdose when using substances containing illicit fentanyl.

Other important factors influencing the clinical effect of an opioid besides potency include half-life and route of administration. Typically, short-acting opioids have a more rapid onset and decay, which can be useful in treating acute pain, but can frequently create a pattern of unstable levels of drug when dosed repeatedly, resulting in both positive and negative reinforcement driving continued use. Moreover, use of short-acting opioids leads to more rapid neuroadaptation, or CNS sensitization/homeostasis, whereby the stronger the opioid and the more rapidly it reaches the brain, the greater the neuroadaptive response [26]. This neuroadaptation is what leads to development of tolerance and physiologic dependence, which tend to occur much earlier with short-acting opioids than with longer-acting opioids.

Longer-acting opioids are typically used only in chronic rather than acute pain. Many such drugs are simply "extended-release" versions of short-acting opioids with an insoluble substance matrix that delays intestinal absorption and metabolism. Others, such as methadone and buprenorphine, are long-acting by design, primarily due to their high affinity for the opioid receptor. Though long-acting opioids may not be quite as reinforcing as short-acting opioids, clinicians should not assume that they are safer or less addictive than short-acting opioids. Importantly, long-acting opioids such as the prior version of Oxycontin™ were commonly tampered with by misusers to instantly produce high levels of the short-acting form of the drug, oxycodone. Abuse-deterrent extended-release formulations have helped to curb this widespread misuse technique (Oxycontin was reformulated in 2010), but not all available long-acting opioids have this technology. Notably, long-acting formulations have been associated with higher rates of overdose, in part due to the above, as well as the fact that combining a long-acting opioid with a CNS depressant such as alcohol or a prescription sedative may be more likely to produce a lengthier and therefore deadlier respiratory depression effect. Even without a second substance, accumulated dosing of long-acting opioids taken at higher levels of frequency than prescribed presents elevated overdose risk, particularly at the initiation stage of use. It typically takes roughly 5 half-lives of a long-acting drug to achieve steady-state in the circulation, which amounts to five full days with methadone, and patients who are impatient to achieve either pain relief or euphoric effect may increase dosing frequency before steady state is reached and before protective tolerance to the drug has begun [27].

2.3 The role of opioids in the treatment of chronic pain

Regarding the controversial therapeutic value of opioids in the treatment of chronic non-cancer pain, there is very little high-quality research evidence. In a widely publicized 2018 JAMA study known as the SPACE trial, done in a Minnesota Veterans population, opioid-naïve patients with chronic back pain, or hip or knee osteoarthritis, were placed on a 12-months period of medication management and randomized to either opioid or non-opioid medications. The primary outcome was pain-related function, measured via Brief Pain Inventory scale; secondary outcomes were pain intensity and medication-related symptoms. The trial results showed no difference between the two groups in pain-related function, lower pain intensity in the non-opioid group, and more common adverse medication-related symptoms in the opioid group. The authors concluded that treatment with opioids was not superior to treatment with non-opioid medications for improving pain-related function over 12 months for moderate to severe chronic back pain or hip or knee osteoarthritis pain [28].

There are other views in the literature more favorable to the appropriate use of prescription opioids for chronic non-cancer pain, particularly in the current context of the ongoing escalation of overdose deaths driven primarily by the use of illicit opioids rather than prescription opioids. In a 2021 analytic review of evidence, Nadeau argued that restricting physicians from prescribing opioids for reasonable indications is a "failed strategy", opining that it was "pill mill" clinics rather than the average medical provider that was responsible for flooding much of the country with large supplies of prescription opioids, prior to a widespread law enforcement crackdown [25]. These clinics not only provided voluminous quantities of opioids, but they also delivered substandard care without appropriate support and supervision, which exacerbated the risk of misuse, diversion, and development of substance use disorders. These effects were prevalent not only in places with large local pill mill distribution networks, but also in more remote areas that were perhaps more susceptible to the lure of opioids because of poverty, mental illness, hopelessness, and other psychosocial factors [29]. According to Nadeau, well-designed studies have demonstrated that the annual case fatality rate attributable to prescribed opioids >100 mg daily morphine-equivalent dose (MED) is in the vicinity of 0.25% per year, which is similar to the risk of death from anticoagulation for stroke prophylaxis for a patient with atrial fibrillation. The twin crisis of high-impact chronic pain, which as noted affects approximately 20 million US adults and an estimated 30% of adults worldwide, necessitates a balanced approach. It remains unclear, however, whether future studies of the effectiveness of long-term use of opioids to ameliorate pain and improve functioning will support or refute the arguments of those who advocate for loosening current restrictions on the prescription of opioids for chronic pain.

Prescription opioid misuse is defined as use of the opioid "in any way other than how the provider directed the use, including greater amount, greater frequency, greater duration, using it for an effect other than intended, using someone else's medication, or using via unauthorized route of administration" [30]. In a 2017 "review of reviews" on chronic pain and opioid misuse, the prevalence of chronic non-cancer pain in individuals known to be misusing prescription opioids is estimated at 48–60%, which is substantially higher than the prevalence of chronic pain in the general population (11–19%) [31]. This finding highlights chronic pain as a major driver of opioid misuse. Reviews were noted to be commonly compromised by limitations including inconsistencies, imprecision, and lack of standardized assessment instruments and definitions of SUD, misuse, addiction, and abuse. They cited an overall lack of high-quality evidence on prevalence, risk factors, optimal clinical assessment, and treatment approaches related to co-occurring chronic pain and substance misuse.

2.4 Opioid use disorder vs. prescription opioid dependence

Development of physiologic dependence on a substance should be viewed as distinct from the development of a substance use disorder (SUD) as defined by DSM-5. Tolerance to a substance is typically expected with prolonged use, and withdrawal symptoms upon cessation of the substance are also part and parcel of physiologic dependence, even without aberrant drug-taking behavior, misuse, craving, or other behavioral components more consistent with substance use disorder [32].

Patients who fall into the category of longtime users of prescription opioids for pain who have developed associated tolerance, physiologic dependence, and fear of physical and emotional distress and withdrawal symptoms when presented with the idea of tapering, have been classified as having a variant of dependence to opioids called complex persistent opioid dependence [33]. This is a distinct phenomenon from opioid use disorder. It is also distinct from simple persistent opioid dependence, in which the patient may have developed tolerance and physiologic dependence but does not approach the idea of tapering or dose adjustment with the degree of fear and/or resistance as does the patient with complex persistent opioid dependence. Given the sheer volume of patients classifiable in one of these two categories, providers in the era of the opioid crisis have been faced with the challenge of how to safely and humanely help them reduce their opioid usage, if/when indeed that is an appropriate and patient-centered goal to pursue. As noted previously, there are significant known harms that can come to patients for whom tapers have been non-consensual, overly rapid, and/or unskillfully executed [7].

3. Screening chronic pain patients for risk of opioid misuse and other substance use

3.1 Factors that contribute to opioid misuse and examples of validated screening tools

Given the need to balance the risks and benefits of use of opioids for chronic pain, how do we select who should receive an opioid prescription in any given clinical scenario? One key aspect of the answer lies in the determination of relative risk of misuse of the prescribed drug, which is dependent on multiple factors: drug factors, provider factors, and patient factors [34].

3.1.1 Drug factors

The relative degree of euphoric or reinforcing effect of a drug depends primarily on the rapidity of its onset of action, and secondarily on both its potency and its half-life. The more quickly a substance reaches the brain and causes dopamine release, the more abuse potential and street value it tends to have.

3.1.2 Provider factors

If the first wave of the opioid crisis taught us anything, it is that most health care providers receive inadequate training in the appropriate prescribing of controlled substances, particularly in scenarios involving acute or chronic pain, anxiety and depression, insomnia, and substance use disorders [23]. The American Medical Association (AMA) has classified these practitioner-based inadequacies as to the "4 D's" (to which 2 additional have subsequently been added):

- **Dated practitioners** whose knowledge of best patient care practices is out of date, leading to inappropriate prescribing choices.

- **Deceived or Duped practitioners** are easily misled by drug-seeking patients who report symptoms or conditions indicating an accepted indication for a controlled substance.

- **Disabled practitioners** have their own psychiatric or medical issues, which may include a substance use disorder, and impair their judgment regarding appropriate prescribing and monitoring.

- **Dishonest practitioners** are typically motivated to prescribe controlled substances by the money they will obtain with this practice; this group is thought to be quite rare in the overall current provider population but during the heyday of "pill mill" clinics, numbers were likely greater.

- **Defiant practitioners** believe they have greater knowledge or expertise than others in a specific practice area and practice in ways that are not supported by evidence on the topic.

- **Distracted practitioners** are overwhelmed by patient care, documentation, and administrative duties and are inadequately attentive to providing safe care and monitoring for patients whom they are treating with controlled substances.

3.1.3 Patient factors

There will always be a proportion of patients who misuse prescription opioids and other controlled drugs for non-medical purposes or will divert them to others for intended profit or for non-medical use. However, it is incumbent upon the modern practitioner to use validated screening tools to try to mitigate and avoid contributing to these potential behaviors when considering initiating the prescription of a controlled substance, and at regular intervals such as every 1–2 years for those using them in a stable and responsible fashion. Specific validated tools and questionnaires are easy to implement in clinical practice and can be filled out by the patient as they wait in the exam room for the practitioner to start the visit. It should be noted that these questionnaires rely on honest self-reporting by the patient, an inherent limitation on reliability. Commonly used validated tools include the following:

- **Pain Medication Questionnaire**: 26-item survey that predicts future opioid misuse and stratifies patients into low, medium, and high risk. It has been validated with good sensitivity and specificity [34].

- **Screener and Opioid Assessment for Patients with Pain-Revised** (SOAPP-R) and **Common Opioid Misuse Measure** (COMM) were cited in a large systematic review to be helpful in the treatment of chronic pain for patients who are either already on long-term opioid therapy and being assessed for recent behavior (COMM), or who are being considered for potential initiation of opioid therapy (SOAPP-R) [34].

- **Opioid Risk Tool**: designed to predict which patients who are prescribed opioids will develop aberrant drug-taking behaviors. Developed in 2005, a 2013 study did not validate its predictive capability [35].

As the COVID-19 pandemic ushered in a sudden and widespread adoption of telemedicine by necessity, the care of patients being prescribed controlled substances was immediately transformed. The use of these screening tools may assist providers with determination of which patients are appropriate for continued support with telemedicine, and which require assessment in clinic with appropriate thorough risk assessment including physical exam, urine toxicology screening, pill count, or other measures not accessible via telehealth [36].

3.2 Assessment of overdose risk and use of naloxone

It is prudent to consider any patient using prescription drugs with the potential to cause overdose to be at some risk of such an outcome, even when that risk is relatively low. For patients considered to be at greater than low risk, proactive prescription of naloxone to mitigate the risk of overdose is the current standard of care and is endorsed by the AMA, CDC, and many other influential public health organizations [37].

To better assess overdose risk, Zedler and colleagues developed a new tool first presented in 2015, called the Risk Index for Overdose or Severe Opioid-induced Respiratory Depression, or RIOSORD, which has been validated in a veteran population of almost two million patients. It contains 17 questions, with a maximum score of 115. Included in the assessment are questions regarding history of psychiatric disorder, presence of pulmonary or liver disease, use of an extended-release opioid, concurrent use of a benzodiazepine or antidepressant, daily morphine equivalent dose (MED), and any recent hospitalizations or emergency department visits [38].

Naloxone is an opioid receptor antagonist and will reverse the respiratory depressant effect of opioids [9]. There are multiple formulations of naloxone which vary by route of administration (intranasal, intramuscular, or intravenous), cost, and shelf life. All are highly effective, and many states offer access to naloxone without a prescription.

As previously noted, screening tools are imperfect and will fail to identify some individuals who will develop aberrant drug-related behaviors. These tools are not a substitute for common sense and good clinical judgment over time. However, they do contribute to the enhancement of patient safety, patient-provider trust, and risk mitigation for patients prescribed or being considered for opioid therapy for treatment of chronic pain.

4. Diagnosis and treatment of opioid use disorder or other SUD in the setting of co-occurring chronic pain

4.1 Approach to the patient

Patients presenting for care who are suffering from chronic pain and/or SUD must be evaluated with thoroughness, compassion, empathy, and respect. A successful clinical approach typically involves reflective listening, acknowledgment and validation of the patient's feelings, absence of judgment, evident expertise, and use of gentle persuasion for the patient to choose to pursue collaborative and volitional change. Motivational interviewing is one evidence-based technique in which patients are encouraged to consider change without confrontation or power struggle, where the provider will "roll with resistance" expressed by the patient, and instead focus on the patient's strengths while projecting optimism regarding their ability to change with proper support [39, 40].

As noted in the previous section, screening tools can be useful in identifying SUD or potential prescription drug misuse, investigating potential mental health comorbidities, and providing a periodic ongoing reassessment of the plan of care. These ideally can be reviewed along with other relevant patient data either before or during the first consultation visit. A thorough patient history is essential for accurate diagnosis and development of a safe and appropriate treatment plan [41, 42]. Ideally, the practitioner will obtain a good understanding of the patient's subjective symptoms and they are established underlying or co-occurring diagnoses, and a detailed understanding of past and current treatment, including medication management, non-pharmacologic interventions, and self-care practices. As above, the clinical approach to gather history should be non-judgmental and empathetic.

The physical exam is a compulsory, standard-of-care component of a medical evaluation for any new patient, and patients presenting with chronic pain and/or SUD histories are no exception. Naturally, a problem-focused exam of the area(s) of the body where pain symptoms are localized will contribute to the diagnosis, and assessment of symptom severity and functional limitations. For patients with concern for SUD, examination of the skin for evidence of injection sites, both old and more recent, can be illuminating, though, in the era of illicit fentanyl, drug smoking has replaced intravenous use in some locales. Evidence of advanced liver disease may manifest as icteric sclerae, jaundiced skin, or abdominal ascites. Poor dentition can be a marker of a variety of SUD-related factors but is particularly common with regular use of methamphetamine. The presence of lymphadenopathy in a patient with SUD may be indicative of an immunocompromised state due to HIV, tuberculosis, or other infectious diseases. A thorough neurologic and mental status examination is also critical to establish neurocognitive and behavioral status, motor and/or sensory deficits, and cranial nerve functioning.

Laboratory tests can be helpful in assessing the presence and severity of organ diseases such as liver and kidney functioning, along with evaluation of relevant metabolic, infectious, hemodynamic, hormonal, and other data. Urine toxicology screening is a standard method of evaluating adherence to expectations around the use of prescribed medications and confirming absence of use of unauthorized substances. Imaging tests are often useful in working up musculoskeletal, gastrointestinal, or CNS complaints. Other useful data can typically be found in the electronic health record, such as other practitioners' assessments, as well as easy access to review of the state prescription monitoring program database, which provides evidence for use of prescribed medications and any detection of unreported use of other controlled prescription medications.

4.2 Reaching a diagnosis and formulating a treatment plan

Substance use disorders are diagnosed using the standardized definition provided in the Diagnostic and Statistical Manual of Mental Disorders, 5th edition (DSM-5), which contains 11 criteria [26]. Diagnosis is classified as mild with a score of 2–3, moderate with a score of 4–5, and severe with a score of 6 or more. It is important to clarify whether the patient's substance use has the potential to have reached a state of physiologic dependence and/or withdrawal with repeated use and attempted cessation, so that management of withdrawal can be prioritized in the earliest stages of treatment.

There is no single treatment or approach that is appropriate for all patients in all scenarios. Treatment planning should always involve a "menu of options" that is considered in a collaborative fashion in consultation with the patient. Ideally, treatment choices will be informed and supported by other stakeholders such as the patient's loved ones and other members of their care team.

For patients with chronic pain who may have developed OUD, treatment options include the following:

- Tapering of medication without other treatment. This course of care will not only fail to provide any therapeutic benefit, but it could also result in the patient seeking relief from drugs obtained from unauthorized sources which, in the era of ubiquitous illicit fentanyl, is acutely life-threatening.

- Tapering followed by treatment with opioid antagonist (naltrexone).

- Treatment with buprenorphine in the outpatient clinic.

- Referral to an opioid treatment program (OTP) for opioid agonist treatment with methadone or buprenorphine.

- Referral to short- or longer-term residential SUD treatment, with the potential to initiate medication for opioid use disorder (MOUD).

Regardless of the specifics of the treatment approach, all patients who have been identified as misusing prescribed medications or otherwise engaging in unhealthy substance use are deserving of the medical provider's concern and attention. The clinical circumstances should be viewed as a therapeutic opportunity to intervene in an impactful and potentially life-saving way.

4.3 Medications for opioid use disorder (MOUD) and their potential utility in the patient with co-occurring chronic pain

There have been many studies confirming the effectiveness and first-line status of MOUD in the treatment of OUD [24, 43]. Interactions between patients with OUD and the medical system, whether in an emergency department, hospital unit, primary care office, or specialty clinic should whenever possibly include prescription of MOUD coupled with timely, logistically feasible follow-up.

4.3.1 Buprenorphine

A semi-synthetic derivative of thebaine developed in the 1980s as an analgesic, buprenorphine is a complex and commonly misunderstood opioid. In the United States, the sublingual formulation was approved by the Food and Drug Administration (FDA) in 2002 for the indication of treatment of opioid dependence (DSM-4 equivalent of opioid use disorder). Its use was limited by restrictions placed on potential prescribers, who were mandated to undergo formal education and training along with application and official authorization by the Drug Enforcement Agency (DEA) to legally prescribe buprenorphine for OUD. These restrictions, which were intended to prevent diversion of the drug, have resulted in a persistently low percentage of available prescribers relative to candidates for use, and a resultant catastrophic unmet need. Further, the implications of these restrictions have led many practitioners to falsely conclude that learning to prescribe buprenorphine is cumbersome, difficult, and better left to others, such as addiction specialists. Tragically, as noted above, at least 80% of individuals with OUD receive no treatment. Ironically, buprenorphine is an extremely safe opioid, indeed safer than not only all other reasonably potent opioids but also many non-opioid medications that all practitioners who treat pain commonly prescribe. Currently, as of the writing of this chapter, there is legislation pending in the US Congress that would remove restrictions on the prescription of buprenorphine for the treatment of OUD.

Buprenorphine's pharmacology includes highly potent mu-opioid receptor (MOR) activity, at least 50 times the analgesic potency of morphine, along with kappa-opioid receptor antagonist activity and delta-opioid receptor agonist activity. Buprenorphine's antagonism at the kappa opioid receptor contributes to an anti-depressant effect, as well as contributing to its ability to diminish and resolve tolerance and hyperalgesia resulting from prolonged use of other opioids. Its delta agonism may contribute to additional analgesia. Its primary metabolite, norbuprenorphine, is unable to cross the blood-brain barrier, which therefore mitigates overdose risk, as brain stem opioid receptors are spared; the opioid receptors in the reward circuitry/limbic system are also spared, which is why buprenorphine can be given to patients with OUD and there is no reinforcing effect. Due to this combination of high potency, excellent safety profile, and lack of psychoactive effect, buprenorphine evolved from its origins as an analgesic to become a first-line treatment for opioid use disorder.

The utility of buprenorphine in the treatment of chronic pain is even more under-appreciated and misunderstood. Due to the above-described legal restrictions, the marketing of the sublingual formulation as a treatment for OUD, and knowledge gaps around its pharmacology, many practitioners are unaware of the advantages of buprenorphine as a medication for patients with chronic pain who require or benefit from a long-acting opioid [44]. There are multiple formulations of buprenorphine that can be used effectively as an analgesic, including transdermal buprenorphine, which was approved in 2010; buccal buprenorphine (brand name Belbuca), approved in 2015; and the sublingual formulation, described above and still approved for the treatment of OUD and not pain, even though buprenorphine's analgesic effects are dose-dependent, and the sublingual formulation is the most potent of any of them. One of the common misconceptions around buprenorphine's pharmacology is that there is a "ceiling effect" for analgesia. In fact, the existence of a ceiling effect pertains specifically and exclusively to respiratory depression, but not to analgesia, which is dose-dependent [45].

4.3.2 Methadone

Methadone is an older synthetic opioid analgesic developed in Germany and introduced in the US in 1947 [46]. It was first described in the treatment of opioid (heroin) addiction in 1965 [47]. It has complex pharmacology, particularly with respect to its long and variable half-life (about 24 hours) and pharmacokinetic properties which, combined with its high potency, pose a significant risk of harm when prescribed by providers less well-versed in best practices around its use, or when it is misused. Due to the delicate nature of initiation of methadone and conversion to stable dosing following transition from other opioids, it has been suggested that only health care providers experienced with this process should undergo this task [48].

For treatment of OUD, since its inception in this context, methadone has been federally regulated and required to be dispensed in a licensed opioid treatment program (OTP), rather than in a typical medical office setting. This is one major practical distinguishing feature from buprenorphine. Many OTP facilities provide not only the medication, which is dispensed daily on-site in liquid formulation, but also support services such as counseling, medical care, and complementary treatment such as acupuncture. For these reasons, methadone's utility in current OUD treatment remains strong, particularly for individuals who benefit from the more rigid structure and robust support of the OTP setting.

Methadone poses significant and unique risk factors within the opioid class, however. It exhibits large inter-individual variation in both bioavailability and elimination half-life. Further, there is a major disconnect between its analgesic effect of only about 6–12 hours, contrasted with half-life of up to 59 hours. Patients will sometimes make the dangerous mistake of taking more than instructed as they are trying to get stabilized during initiation. Each dose's respiratory depressant effect can last up to several days and is cumulative over regular dosing, so too high a starting dose, or overuse of the prescribed dose, is particularly problematic during this early phase before the drug has reached a steady state, which normally takes about five days. Methadone is particularly risky for patients co-prescribed or otherwise using benzodiazepines or other CNS depressants, conferring additional overdose risk. Lastly, particularly at higher doses, methadone can prolong the QT interval on an electrocardiogram (ECG) which is a sign of potential cardiac arrest. It is prudent to check a baseline ECG before methadone is initiated. Some have suggested checking again at 50 mg, 100 mg, and any incremental increase of 20 mg thereafter, though there is no clear consensus [48].

Methadone does offer some attractive pharmacologic advantages as a potent long-acting opioid analgesic compared to other options. It is an N-methyl-d-aspartate (NMDA) receptor antagonist as well as a serotonin-norepinephrine reuptake inhibitor, which together may contribute to its anti-hyperalgesic effect after transitioning from other opioids, as well as its reputation for effectiveness in neuropathic pain syndromes [48].

4.3.3 Naltrexone

Developed in the 1970s, naltrexone is a long-acting competitive antagonist at opioid receptors with the capacity to block the subjective and objective effects of opioids [49]. It is an effective antagonist at mu- and kappa-opioid receptors, less so at the delta subtype. It is thought to block glutamate and may contribute to reduction in craving for and protracted withdrawal from alcohol through that mechanism.

Oral naltrexone was approved by the FDA in 1984 for "blockade of the effects of exogenously administered opioids" [49]. It is also approved for alcohol use disorder. Its onset is rapid, reaching peak plasma level within 1 hour, and has a relatively brief half-life of 4 hours. It is metabolized by the liver and severe liver impairment may be an obstacle to use.

An extended-release, injectable formulation of naltrexone was approved in 2006 first for treatment of alcohol use disorder, with opioid use disorder following in 2010. It is administered intramuscularly in the gluteal region, and is typically well-tolerated, particularly with a period of several days of use of oral naltrexone prior to injection [49]. The most common adverse effects are injection site pain, nausea, other gastrointestinal upset, or flu-like symptoms. The formulation contains 380 mg of naltrexone, releasing levels of 1 ng/mL or above for a period of 4–5 weeks, without the need to adjust the dose for weight, age, health status, or other factors.

Studies comparing the effectiveness of ER-naltrexone (XR-NTX) and buprenorphine-naloxone (BUP-NX) for the treatment of opioid use disorder have been performed. In the "X:BOT" study, a multicenter, open-label randomized controlled trial published in 2018 and funded by the National Institutes of Drug Abuse (NIDA) Clinical Trials Network, the 2 medications were found to be equally safe and effective once initiated [50]. Some patients had more difficulty with initiation of XR-NTX compared to BUP-NX, which was in part due to a lack of formal optimization and uniformity of induction and withdrawal protocols between testing sites, of which there were 8 around the country. Authors concluded that the research community should prioritize improving XR-NTX induction and retention strategies. In a more recent study published in JAMA in 2022, however, Xu and colleagues importantly found that buprenorphine outperformed naltrexone in the category of decreasing overdose risk [51].

Naltrexone in compounded oral formulation has been used in the context of chronic pain in the form of "low dose naltrexone" for treatment of CNS-mediated generalized pain syndromes such as fibromyalgia, inflammatory bowel conditions, or multiple sclerosis. Dosing is generally in the range of 4–5 mg daily, whereas daily dose for treatment of OUD is 50 mg. It is thought to work as a modulator of glial cells and inflammatory chemicals in the CNS. It was systematically reviewed in 2020 with favorable findings suggesting a need for further investigation and increased clinical use [52].

Patients may find it difficult to know which of the 3 above-described medications approved for OUD to choose, particularly in the context of chronic pain. Although individual cases will vary, generally it would not be advisable to choose naltrexone for patients with the following circumstances:

- At high risk for overdose
- Have not tolerated extended periods of opioid abstinence in past attempts
- Have tended to experience protracted and severe withdrawal symptoms following cessation of opioids
- Have unstable psychiatric symptoms
- Level of chronic pain requires or is currently being treated with opioids
- Have advanced liver disease, impending liver failure, or acute hepatitis

Whichever of these evidence-based treatment options is ultimately pursued, it is critical that patients are carefully matched to the best MOUD treatment for their specific circumstances and needs, then monitored and supported to optimize stability in the patient-provider relationship to foster best outcomes.

4.4 Other medications useful in co-occurring chronic pain and SUD

In the management of chronic pain, typically a combination of agents is prescribed to provide analgesia using different neurochemical pathways [17]. Opioids should be used only when other non-opioid medications, and non-pharmacologic pain management strategies, have failed to adequately address pain severity and associated functional impairment [6]. Patients with active SUD, and/or a personal or family history thereof, should even more pointedly be recommended to avoid controlled substances which may trigger unhealthy substance use in a manner that is unsafe and counterproductive to the goals of treatment. Examples of commonly used non-opioid medications include the following [17]:

- **Non-steroidal anti-inflammatory drugs (NSAIDs):** these are the most widely used analgesics, indicated for mid to moderate somatic pain, and used often in combination with opioids for severe pain. They work by inhibiting prostaglandin production, thereby reducing the sensitization of peripheral nerves, and curbing the inflammatory response. Most common adverse effects include gastrointestinal symptoms, renal toxicity, and inhibition of platelet functioning leading to an increased risk of bleeding.
- **Antidepressants:** include older agents such as tricyclic antidepressants, and newer selective serotonin and norepinephrine reuptake inhibitors (SNRIs). Tricyclic agents are considered first-line treatment for neuropathic pain such as diabetic neuropathy, with the greatest potency in amitriptyline, imipramine, and doxepin, and less effective but also fewer anticholinergic adverse effects with nortriptyline and desipramine. SNRIs include duloxetine, which is approved by the FDA for fibromyalgia and is considered a first-line drug for patients with chronic low back pain by the American College of Physicians, along with venlafaxine.
- **Anticonvulsants**: this class has been used widely in the treatment of neuropathic pain and other dysesthesia pain syndromes characterized by burning or lancinating pain. Gabapentin has been commonly prescribed, along with pregabalin,

both of which are approved for diabetic peripheral neuropathy and post-herpetic neuralgia, the latter also approved for fibromyalgia. Carbamazepine, valproic acid, and other agents have been used effectively for paroxysmal facial pain and headache syndromes. All medications in this category have potential for significant adverse effects and tolerability issues.

- **Muscle relaxants**: this category includes several classes of medications with a variety of mechanisms of action, some of which are poorly understood. All tend to have significant sedating effects due to primarily CNS-mediated activity, which may limit daytime use. Use at bedtime may assist with insomnia along with overnight pain control in appropriate patients.

- **Topical agents**: a variety of agents are available which can be applied locally to painful areas when symptoms are focal. These include topical diclofenac, an NSAID; lidocaine transdermal patches or lidocaine-based ointment, gel or cream, a local anesthetic; capsaicin, a naturally-occurring extract from cayenne pepper which inhibits substance P and is useful for neuropathic pain after initial worsening of burning symptoms; products now available in many states containing formulations of cannabinoid-derived salves, creams, gels and ointments; and other options available over-the-counter in pharmacies such as camphor-based and menthol-based counterirritants.

5. Non-pharmacologic pain management modalities

In approaching a patient with co-occurring chronic pain and SUD, it is important for the clinician to recognize the multiple functional domains affected: body, brain (CNS), mind, and spirit. Structural and functional changes in the brain have been well-documented and contribute to reorganization of neural networks involved in behavior, emotional regulation, identity formation, and capacity for enjoyment of life. Thinking may be distorted due to chronically focused attention on pain and distress signals, frequently attached to drug-related cues, which biases thoughts and attitudes toward negative, maladaptive patterns of fear, avoidance, catastrophizing, and disengagement. Treatment modalities aimed at improving self-efficacy and coping skills are critical in achieving good outcomes. Below are some categories and examples of such approaches.

Special mention is given to the existence and strong evidence in favor of structured interdisciplinary pain rehabilitation programs [53]. Though not commonly found, these programs provide holistic care to a cohort of patients and typically include medical management, psychological counseling, movement-based therapy, and relaxation training. They are often managed by a nurse or allied health provider. The team of specialists communicates about each patient in the program in a longitudinal and coordinated fashion to optimize individual patient progress and outcomes, emphasizing training the patient in sustainable self-care techniques.

5.1 Movement-based therapies

Ref. [54] At a basic level, exercise and movement are helpful and adaptive for patients with chronic pain, many of whom have developed kinesiophobia, or fear of movement. Physical therapy is often a helpful first step in addressing that fear and gradually improving activity tolerance. Occupational therapy assesses and intervenes to maintain or re-establish meaningful activities or occupations specific to a patient's circumstances, such as working in an office environment or providing care to small children. Tai chi is an evidence-based form of ancient Chinese movement, breathing, and harnessing of energy (chi) that has been used widely in chronic pain treatment, especially in interdisciplinary chronic pain rehabilitation programs. Yoga is another validated technique for combining anaerobic exercise, breathing, mindfulness, and energy movement, and has become very popular both in chronic pain treatment and as an approach for general wellness.

5.2 Bodywork treatments

Ref. [54] Acupuncture is an ancient Chinese technique using specific needle placement, with available modern innovations such as the use of percutaneous electrical nerve stimulation, which has been shown to be effective for a variety of chronic pain conditions, including headache syndromes, chronic low back pain, and other common structural and functional pain syndromes. Chiropractic treatment aims to realign structural abnormalities via manual manipulation of the spine, with evidence most positive for low back pain and less so for neck and upper back pain. Osteopathic manipulation therapy (OMT) similarly uses structural manipulation techniques but in contrast to chiropractic care, OMT is not exclusively focused on the spine as a site for application of gentle pressure on body tissues. Massage therapy is performed by trained, licensed providers using various styles ranging from very gentle to deep tissue techniques, with the goal of reduction of muscle tension as well as general relaxation of body and mind. It has been shown in a host of studies to be useful in chronic pain [55].

5.3 Psychosocial treatment for chronic pain

Ref. [54] Enhancing insight into the role of a patient's thoughts, emotions, and behaviors on functional capacity and subjective level of pain is of paramount importance and may be approached with specific counseling techniques, which are often provided by mental health specialists but may also be used by medical providers such as pain or addiction medicine specialists, or primary care providers [56]. Motivational interviewing is a patient-centered approach that encourages the patient to undergo behavior change in a manner consistent with their own choice and empowerment. Cognitive restructuring aims to increase a patient's awareness of maladaptive thoughts and behavioral patterns and encourages replacing those with more positive, adaptive ones. Cognitive-behavioral therapy (CBT) is a broad category of a well-studied treatment that, like cognitive restructuring, emphasizes the pursuit of change in maladaptive thoughts and behaviors. Emphasis is on improvement of coping skills, reducing fear of movement and activity, development of techniques for relaxation and enjoyment, and establishing adaptive routines. Acceptance-Commitment Therapy (ACT) is a modification of CBT that emphasizes cognitive flexibility and encourages non-judgmental detachment from the experience of pain, with the goal to engage in meaningful and rewarding activities despite the presence of pain.

5.4 Self-directed non-pharmacologic management of chronic pain

Self-management of chronic pain is a vital component of a successful pain management approach. It is often impractical at best to access the full gamut of evidence-based professional treatment, due to both availability and cost; moreover, self-care tends to enhance the patient's sense of autonomy, self-reliance, and self-efficacy while incorporating activities and techniques that are consistent with the patient's belief system. The following are examples of self-care approaches:

- **Mindfulness-based Stress Reduction** (MBSR): developed by Jon Kabat-Zinn in his 1990 book Full Catastrophe Living, MBSR is an 8-week evidence-based course offered in hundreds of medical settings and teaches a Buddhist-influenced style of mindfulness meditation practice, along with body scanning and certain yoga postures. It promotes a non-judgmental uncoupling of the sensory aspects of pain from its emotional evaluative dimensions. It has been studied extensively in the context of chronic pain and has been shown to be equally effective and more cost-effective than CBT provided professionally [57].

- **Spirituality**: engagement in prayer and faith-based activity has been shown to facilitate well-being and contribute positively to the management of chronic pain [58].

- **Exercise**: an essential component of a comprehensive approach to pain management, exercise may be part of a prescribed movement treatment such as physical therapy, or may involve less structured, patient-directed activity. It is acknowledged that while individualized exercise therapy generally enhances functional outcomes, there are limitations to the level of intensity and duration of activity that a given patient attempt if exacerbations in pain and both physical and psychological setbacks are to be avoided. In general, exercise should be approached gradually and increased incrementally. Aquatic therapy, such as walking in a warm pool, can be a good first step [59].

- **Sleep hygiene**: sleep disorders are among the most common comorbidities for those experiencing chronic pain [60]. Sleep medications are commonly prescribed, and though these may be of benefit, it is appropriate for practitioners to emphasize sleep hygiene improvement for more effective and sustainable results. Examples of recommended aspects of sleep hygiene include sticking with a sleep/wake schedule, not eating too close to bedtime and avoiding evening foods that are difficult to digest or cause reflux, creating a "bedtime ritual", limiting daytime napping, and engaging in routine daily physical activity.

- **Nutrition** is both a "mainstream" and complementary/integrative component of a well-rounded chronic pain management approach. Of course, eating a healthy, balanced diet with avoidance of overeating or restrictive eating patterns is advisable. The use of dietary supplements in pain management has not been supported by evidence, according to the National Center for Complementary and Integrative Health (NCCIH, an agency of the National Institutes of Health). Obesity is a known risk factor for spinal degenerative disc disease, and osteoarthritis of the lower back, hips, and knees [61].

- **Peer support groups:** there are available online and in-person meetings for patients suffering from a range of chronic pain conditions such as fibromyalgia, lupus, irritable bowel syndrome, sickle cell disease, and many others [62]. In addition, there are 12-step "pain recovery" books that focus on the intersection of pain and substance use disorders, using the model and framework that has been so critical and well-trod by individuals who have participated in Alcoholics Anonymous or Narcotics Anonymous programs.

6. Interventional procedures used in chronic pain management

A variety of procedural management options are available for patients with chronic pain, with a range of techniques and associated therapeutic effects [63].

- **Trigger point injections**: local injection of anesthetic into focally tender areas of muscle and soft tissue known as "trigger points" can produce short-term relief for both acute and chronic myofascial pain conditions. Controversy exists as to what agent should be injected and how often. Dry needling may concurrently or alternatively be employed, and both acupuncture and physical therapy may be useful adjunctive approaches. Techniques for this approach were described in depth by Dr. Janet Travell, physician to President John F Kennedy, in her seminal 1983 text on myofascial pain [64].

- **Local neural blockade**: can be used for both diagnostic and therapeutic purposes. Commonly used on the medial branch nerves at spinal facet joints, if pain relief is greater than 80%, patients may be candidates for radiofrequency nerve ablation (neurotomy) at that level, with much longer-lasting relief. Recently, peripheral nerves have also been targeted [65].

- **Spinal epidural steroid injections**: used in the treatment of mechanical back and neck pain, with best results typically seen when radiculopathy is present, and when symptoms have been present less than 6 months or are acutely exacerbated [66]; facet blocks are typically used in cases without radicular signs.

- **Sympathetic blockade**: indicated for pain involving the sympathetic nervous system and viscera. Nociceptive input from the upper extremities, head, and neck can be blocked via the stellate ganglion; abdominal visceral pain can be approached by blocking the celiac ganglion, while urogenital visceral is approached via the hypogastric plexus. Lumbar sympathetic ganglia mediate pain in the lower extremities, and blockade may be useful in neuropathic lower extremity pain from failed back surgery syndrome or complex regional pain syndrome of the lower limb [67].

- **Spinal cord stimulation** was first introduced in 1967, but there have been innovations in recent years that have significantly improved the effectiveness of this intervention, in particular for failed back surgery syndrome and peripheral neuropathy. Because it involves surgical implantation, it is generally reserved for patients who have failed more conservative interventional therapies [68].

7. Conclusion

Patients who are living with chronic pain and a history of SUD and are attempting to improve their quality of life and avoid unhealthy substance use are to be credited for their resilience, courage, and perseverance in staying "within the system" and entrusting their care to a team of providers. Often, these patients are the victims of stigma and judgment, experiencing negative interactions with individual providers and with the health care system as a whole. Today's unprecedented levels of fatal drug overdoses necessitate a shift toward harm reduction and toward a willingness to partner with patients whose choices do not always perfectly align with prescribed recommendations, so that we may help them avoid making their last dangerous choice. With the right approach, these patients can be offered safe, effective, holistic care that aims to address the various domains of their suffering, including physical symptoms, emotional distress and trauma, and disengagement from meaningful activity. Best results are generally found when a team of professionals provides coordinated interdisciplinary care. When such care is impractical or unavailable, individual components of evidence-based interventions and approaches can still be pursued with excellent patient-centered results, and with fulfilling, gratifying long-term relationships between patients and providers.

Author details

Gregory Rudolf
Swedish Health Services, Seattle, USA

*Address all correspondence to: gdrudolf@aol.com

References

[1] Ciccarone D. The triple wave epidemic: Supply and demand drivers of the US opioid overdose crisis. The International Journal on Drug Policy. 2019;**71**:183-188

[2] Rudd RA. Increases in Drug and Opioid-Involved Overdose Deaths. Unites States 2010-2015: MMWR; 2015

[3] Bernard SA, Chelminski PR, Ives TJ, et al. Management of pain in the United States—A brief history and implications for the opioid epidemic. Health Services Insights. 2018;**11**:1178632918819440

[4] Van Zee A. The promotion and marketing of oxycontin: Commercial triumph, public health tragedy. American Journal of Public Health. 2009;**99**(2):221-227

[5] International Association for the Study of Pain. The global burden of low back pain: fact sheet. 2021.

[6] Dowell D, Haegerich TM, Chou R. CDC guideline for prescribing opioids for chronic pain- United States, 2016. MMWR - Recommendations and Reports. 2016;**65**(RR-1):1-49

[7] Coffin PO, Barreveld AM. Inherited patients taking opioids for chronic pain- considerations for primary care. The New England Journal of Medicine. 2022;**386**(7):611-613

[8] Grub I, Firemark A, Mayhew M, et al. Taking opioids in times of crisis: Institutional oversight, chronic pain and suffering in an integrated healthcare delivery system in the US. The International Journal on Drug Policy. 2019;**74**:62-68

[9] Mars SG, Bourgois P, Karandinos G, et al. "Every 'never' I ever said came true": Transitions from opioid pills to heron injecting. The International Journal on Drug Policy. 2014;**25**(2):257-266

[10] US Drug Enforcement Administration. National Drug Threat Assessment. 2017b https://www.dea.gov/documents/2017/10/01/2017-national-drug-threat-assessment.

[11] Kalkman GA, van den Brink W, Pierce M, Atsma F, Vissers KCP, et al. Monitoring opioids in Europe: The need for shared definitions and measuring drivers of opioid use and related harms. European Addiction Research. 2022;**28**:231-240

[12] Mills SEE, Nicholson KP, Smith BH. Chronic pain: A review of its epidemiology and associated factors in population-based studies. British Journal of Anaesthesia. 2019;**123**(2):e273-e283

[13] Humphreys KH, Shover CL, Andrews CM, et al. Responding to the opioid crisis in North America and beyond: Recommendations of the Stanford-lancet commission. The Lancet Commissions. 2022;**399**(10324): 555-604

[14] Edlund MJ, Martin BC, Russo JE, et al. The role of opioid prescription in incident opioid abuse and dependence among individuals with chronic noncancer pain. The Clinical Journal of Pain. 2014;**30**(7):557-564

[15] Vos T, Allen C, Arora M, et al. Global, regional, and national incidence, prevalence, and years lived with disability for 328 diseases and injuries for 195 countries, 1995-2016: A systematic analysis for the global burden of disease study 2016. Lancet. 2017;**390**:1211-1259

[16] Karran EL, Grant AR, Moseley GL. Low back pain and the social determinants of health: A systematic review and narrative synthesis. Pain. 2020;**161**:2476-2493

[17] Volkow ND, McLellan AT. Opioid abuse in chronic pain-misconceptions and mitigation strategies. The New England Journal of Medicine. 2016;**374**:1253-1263

[18] Koob GF. Neurobiology of opioid addiction: Opponent process, Hyperkatifeia, and negative reinforcement. Biological Psychiatry. 2020;**87**(1):44-53

[19] Frew AK, Drummond PD. Negative affect, pain, and sex: The role of endogenous opioids. Pain. 2007;**132**(1):S77-S85

[20] Philips K, Clauw DJ. Central pain mechanisms in chronic pain states – Maybe it is all in their head. Best Practice & Research. Clinical Rheumatology. 2011;**25**(2):141-154

[21] Villarroel L, Mardian AS, Timme E, et al. Implementation of the Arizona pain and addiction curriculum: Findings and implications from a statewide evaluation. Frontiers in Public Health. 2021;**9**:731016

[22] Moayedi M, Davis KD. Theories of pain: From specificity to gate control. Journal of Neurophysiology. 2012;**109**(1):5-12

[23] Faulx D, Baldwin J, Zorrah Q, et al. Adverse childhood events in the mental health discussion. American Journal of Public Health. 2011;**101**(7):1156-1157

[24] Cavacuiti C. The pharmacology of opioids. In: Robeck IR, Malinoff HL, et al., editors. The American Society of Addiction Medicine Handbook on Pain and Addiction. New York: Oxford University Press; 2018. pp. 83-95

[25] Nadeau SE, Wu JK, Lawhern RA. Opioids and chronic pain: An analytic review of the clinical evidence. Frontiers Pain Research. 2021;**2**:721357

[26] Diagnostic and Statistical Manual of Mental Disorders. 5th ed. American Psychiatric Association; 2013

[27] National Center for Biotechnology Information. PubChem Compound Summary for CID 62156, Carfentanil. Retrieved May 26, 2022 from https://pubchem.ncbi.nlm.nih.gov/compound/carfentanil

[28] Krebs EE, Gravely A, Nugent S, et al. Effect of opioid vs non-opioid medications on pain-related functioning in patients with chronic back pain or hip or knee osteoarthritis pain. Journal of the American Medical Association. 2018;**319**(9):872-882

[29] Office of the Inspector General. Concerns about opioid use in Medicare part D bin the Appalachian region. US Department of Health and Human Services. 2019 OEI-02-18-00224

[30] NIDA. Prescription opioids DrugFacts. 2021. Retrieved from https://nida.nih.gov/publications/drugfacts/prescription-opioids.

[31] Voon P, Karamouzian M, Kerr T. Chronic pain and opioid misuse: A review of reviews. Substance Abuse Treatment, Prevention, and Policy. 2017;**12**:36

[32] Nestler EJ. Is there a common molecular pathway for addiction? Nature Neuroscience. 2005;**8**(11):1445-1449

[33] Manhapra A, Sullivan M, Ballantyne JC, et al. Complex persistent opioid dependence with long-term opioids: A gray area that needs definition, better understanding,

treatment guidance, and policy changes. Journal of General Internal Medicine. 2020;**35**(Suppl 3):964-971

[34] Lawrence R, Mogford D, Colvin L. Systematic review to determine which validated measurement tools can be used to assess risk of problematic analgesic use in patients with chronic pain. British Journal of Anesthesia. 2017;**119**:1092-1109

[35] Witkin LR, Diskina D, Fernandes S, et al. Usefulness of the opioid risk tool to predict aberrant drug-related behavior in patients receiving opioids for the treatment of chronic pain. Journal of Opioid Management. 2013;**9**(3):177-187

[36] Ogilvie CB, Jotwani R, Joshi J, et al. Review of opioid risk assessment tools with the growing need for telemedicine. Pain Management. 2021;**11**(2):97-100

[37] Robinson A, Wermeling D. Intranasal naloxone administration for treatment of opioid overdose. American Journal of Health-System Pharmacy. 2014;**71**(24):2129-2135

[38] Zedler BK, Saunders WB, Joyce AR, et al. Validation of a screening risk index for serious prescription opioid-induced respiratory depression or overdose in a US commercial health plan claims database. Pain Medicine. 2018;**19**:68-78

[39] Anekar AA, Cascella M. WHO analgesic ladder. (updated 2022 may 15). In: StatPearls (Internet). Treasure Island (FL): StatPearls Publishing; 2022

[40] Bischof G, Bischof A, Rumpf HJ. Motivational interviewing: An evidence-based approach for use in medical practice. Deutsches Ärzteblatt International. 2021;**118**(7):109-115

[41] Longo LP, Parran TV, Johnson B, et al. Addiction, part 2: Identification and management of the drug-seeking patient. American Family Physician. 2006;**61**:2401-2408

[42] Institute of Medicine of the National Academy of Sciences. Relieving Pain in America: A Blueprint for Transforming Prevention, Care, Education and Research. Washington, DC: National Academies Press; 2011

[43] Dupont RL, Parran TV, Wilford BB. Understanding and preventing opioid misuse and abuse. In: Robeck IR, Malinoff HL, et al., editors. The American Society of Addiction Medicine Handbook on Pain and Addiction. New York: Oxford University Press; 2018. pp. 96-111

[44] Rudolf GD. Buprenorphine in the treatment of chronic pain. Physical Medicine and Rehabilitation Clinics of North America. 2020;**31**(2):195-204

[45] Dahan A, Yassen A, Romberg R, et al. Buprenorphine induces ceiling in respiratory depression but not in analgesia. British Journal of Anaesthesia. 2006;**96**(5):627-632

[46] Substance Abuse and Mental Health Services Administration. US Department of Health and Human Services. Treatment Improvement Protocol 63. 2021 PEP21-02-01-002

[47] Ausubel DP. The dole-Nyswander treatment of heroin addiction. Journal of the American Medical Association. 1966;**195**(11):949-950

[48] Kreutzwiser D, Tawfic QA. Methadone for pain management: A pharmacotherapeutic review. CNS Drugs. 2020;**34**(8):827-839

[49] Center for Substance Use Treatment. Incorporating alcohol pharmacotherapies into medical practice. In: Treatment

Improvement Protocol (TIP) 49. Chapter 5: Extended-Release Injectable Naltrexone. Rockville (MD): Substance Abuse and Mental Health Services Administration (US); 2009 Available from: https://www.ncbi.nlm.nih.gov/books/NBK64031

[50] Lee JD, Nunes EV Jr, Novo P, et al. Comparative effectiveness of extended-release naltrexone versus buprenorphine-naloxone for opioid relapse prevention (X:BOT): A multicentre, open-label, randomized controlled trial. Lancet. 2018;**391**(10118):309-318

[51] Xu KY, Mintz CM, Presnall N, et al. Comparative effectiveness associated with buprenorphine and naltrexone in opioid use disorder and co-occurring polysubstance use. JAMA Network Open. 2022;**5**(5):e2211363

[52] Kim PS, Fishman MA. Low dose naltrexone for chronic pain: Update and systematic review. Current Pain and Headache Reports. 2020;**24**(10):64

[53] Gerdle B, Fischer MR, Ringqvist A. Interdisciplinary pain rehabilitation programs: Evidence and clinical real-world results. Pain Management-From Pain Mechanisms to Patient Care. 2022. DOI: 10.5772/intechopen.102411

[54] US Department of Health and Human Services. Pain Management Best Practices Inter-Agency Task Force Report: Updates, Gaps, Inconsistencies, and Recommendations. Retrieved from: https://www.hhs.gov/ash/advisory-committees/pain/reports/index.html

[55] Melzack R. From the gate to the neuromatrix. Pain. 1999;**Suppl 6**:S121-S126

[56] MacCracken LM, Yu L, Vowles KE. New generation psychological treatments in chronic pain. BMJ. 2022;**376**:e057212

[57] Herman PM, Anderson ML, et al. Cost-effectiveness of mindfulness-based stress reduction vs cognitive behavioral therapy or usual care among adults with chronic low back pain. Spine. 2017;**42**(20):1511-1520

[58] Edwards JV, Briggs M, et al. Self-management of chronic pain: The role of religious faith. Journal of Disability and Religion. 2016;**20**(4):291-306

[59] Fisken A, Keogh JW, Waters DL, et al. Perceived benefits, motives, and barriers to aqua-based exercise among older adults with and without osteoarthritis. Journal of Applied Gerontology. 2015;**34**(3):377-396

[60] Davin S, Wilt J, Covington E, et al. Variability in the relationship between sleep and pain in patients undergoing interdisciplinary rehabilitation for chronic pain. Pain Medicine. 2014;**15**(6):1043-1051

[61] Narouze S, Souzdalnitzki D. Obesity and chronic pain: Opportunities for better patient care. Pain Management. 2015;**5**(4):217-219

[62] Rheulm LS, Karoly P, Enders C. A randomized controlled evaluation of an online chronic pain self-management program. Pain. 2012;**153**:319-330

[63] Hoydonckx Y, Kumar P, Flamer D, et al. Quality of chronic pain interventional treatment guidelines from pain societies: Assessment from the AGREE 2 instrument. European Journal of Pain. 2020;**24**(4):704-721

[64] Travell JG, Simon DG. Myofascial Pain and Dysfunction. Baltimore: Williams and Wilkins; 1983

[65] Lee DW, Pritzlaff S, Jung MJ, et al. Latest evidence-based application for radiofrequency neurotomy

(LEARN): Best practice guidelines from the American Society of Pain and Neuroscience (ASPN). Journal of Pain Research. 2021;**14**:2807-2831

[66] Carassiti M, Pascarella G, Strumia A, et al. Epidural steroid injections for low back pain: A narrative review. International Journal of Environmental Research and Public Health. 2021;**19**(1):231

[67] Cheng J, You J, Grille M, et al. Outcomes of sympathetic blocks in the management of complex regional pain syndrome: A retrospective cohort study. Anesthesiology. 2019;**131**:883-893

[68] Eckermann JM, Pilitsis JG, Vannaboutathong MS, et al. Systematic literature review of spinal cord stimulation in patients with chronic back pain without prior spine surgery. Frontiers Pain Research. 18 Aug 2021. DOI: 10.1111/ner.13519

Chapter 3

Quantitative Assessment Methods for the Severity of Drug Dependences and Corresponding Rehabilitation Programs

Mu Wang, Yu-Xiang Qian, Zeng-Hui Ding,
Cun-Feng Yuan, Xian-Jun Yang, Yu Liu and Yi-Ning Sun

Abstract

Drug use is a worldwide issue, and how to treat it is even a greater challenge. It is important for drug dependences to receive interventions and treatments in time. Before receiving treatments, an effective screening or diagnosis assessment is necessary, and patients should have an assessment to understand the severity of drug use–related disorders. For more than 40 years, the instruments to assess the severity of drug dependence have been developed well, and different quantitative methods can cover almost every field of the symptoms in different periods and stages of drug addiction. This chapter reviews more than 20 drug dependence screening and diagnosis assessments and different types of treatments. These quantitative assessments can provide drug dependences a comprehensive diagnosis of their drug use–related disorders. The treatments should be designed for different level of drug dependence. **Core tip:** We reviewed the screening, severity assessments, treatments for drug use–related disorders. The existing screening or severity assessments can provide us a comprehensive diagnosis of the disorders. However, after discussing the treatments, we found that conventional treatments focus more on symptoms amelioration and drug effects reduction. It is necessary to develop personalized and comprehensive treatment based on quantitative assessments.

Keywords: drug dependence, assessments, screening, treatments, exercise

1. Introduction

Drug dependence has become a worldwide issue, and 31 million individuals are suffering from its negative effect [1]. Even worse, according to National Center for Health Statistics, 70,630 people were killed by drug-involved overdose in 2019 [2]. Moreover, yearly economy effect from illicit drug use is around 193 billion dollars in the United States [3]. It is important for drug dependences to receive interventions and treatments in time. Before receiving treatments, an effective screening or diagnosis assessment is necessary [4]. This review covers quantitative assessment methods for drug dependences and the corresponding treatments. It concluded more than 20 quantitative instruments that are put into three main categories, screening, severity diagnosis assessments, and treatment outcomes assessments. In addition, three different types of treatments, conventional treatments, emergency treatments, and novel treatment, are discussed.

2. Assessments

2.1 Screening

Screening instruments usually are brief and easy to conduct. They are considered as "flagging," because it's the fundament of further assessments or treatments [5, 6]. The screening instruments tend to diagnose the presence of potential drug use–related disorders in specific fields, such as psychopathology, physiology, and social ability. The answers of screening questions are usually "yes" or "no."

World Health Organization (WHO) developed The Alcohol, Smoking and Substance Involvement Screening Test (ASSIST) to screen and manage substance use and related issues. ASSIST has eight items to detect more than nine types of substance and scored 0.58–0.90 in test-retest reliability [7, 8]. Brown et al. proposed a two-phase assessment, A Two-item Conjoint Screen for Alcohol and Other Drug Problems (TICS) for screening alcohol and drug disorders [9]. TICS has nine questions in phase 1 and five questions in phase 2. One item's answer is positive or negative, and the rest is never, rarely, sometimes, or often. TICS can screen around 80% drug dependences [9]. There is an approach, named Prenatal Substance Abuse Screen (5Ps), developed for prenatal females. The woman needs treatments if there is a "yes" in any of the five items. The overall accuracy of whether the woman needs treatments in 5Ps 0.776 [10].

Some screening techniques would contain more items to obtain more information. Skinner designed The Drug Abuse Screening Test (DAST), as a screening and treatment evaluation instrument for drug dependences [11]. It has 28 items, including background, drug use history, social stability, and psychology. The answer for each item is "yes" or "no" and scored 1 point for "yes," 0 for "no," except for items 4,5, and 7, for which a "no" response is given a score of "1." The cutoff point is 6 and 12. If the score of a patient is larger than 5 or larger than 11, they will be considered to be "might" or "definitely" have drug use disorders, respectively. The reliability of DAST was 0.86–0.91 in Internal Consistency Reliability [11]. DAST-10 and DAST-20 are two shortened versions of DAST and drug use disorders can be screened faster in these two [12]. Another one is CAGE-adapted to Include Drugs (CAGE-AID) [13]. CAGE is derived from four sections: Cut down, Annoyed, Guilty, and Eye-opener. The result indicates clinical significance, if two or greater questions are "yes" [13]. CAGE-AID had general good to excellent performance in different subjects [14, 15].

2.2 Severity diagnosis assessments

Severity diagnosis assessments are to recognize the drug use–related disorders and estimate the level of the disorders. These assessments contain multiple items and have score for each item. Usually, the higher score represents the greater level of severity. Since 1970s, scientists have been studying on the assessments to diagnose the severity of drug dependence. After 40 years, a number of addiction severity assessments have been developed. Addiction severity index (ASI) is one of the most famous ones. ASI was proposed by A. Thomas McLellan and his colleagues (1980). It is a structured clinical interview, focusing on several areas, including medical status, employment status, alcohol use, drug use, legal status, family relationships, social relationships, and psychological functioning. Higher score in ASI means the higher level of severity and greater indication of accepting treatment [16]. This instrument has been used more than 30 years and is considered as gold standard in measuring the severity of drug addiction. The reliability of ASI has been tested by different studies. For example, both McLellan et al. and Hodgins et al. claim that ASI is generally reliable, and most parts are good to excellent, in addiction severity assessment [17, 18]. Now, ASI has developed into sixth version, ASI-6. There are also several adjusted versions of ASI, such as The Addiction Severity Index, Lite version (ASI-Lite) [19] and Addiction Severity Index self-report form (ASI-SR) [20].

Psychiatric disorders are the main concerned part in drug dependence severity assessments. Some psychological disorders assessments are directly utilized in drug dependence. Diagnostic and Statistical Manual of Mental Disorders (DSM) is an assessment for psychiatric disorders. The first version of DSM, DSM-1, was designed by American Psychiatric Association in 1952, and then it has been adjusted into several versions, DSM-II, DSM-III, DSM-III-R, DSM-IV, DSM-IV-TR, and DSM-5 [21]. Although DSM series were developed to measure mental disorders, they were widely used in drug disorders [22] and as a benchmark or to compare with other drug-dependent severity assessments [23, 24]. DSM series are reliable in drug dependence severity assessments. For example, DSM-5 performed good to excellent in alcohol, opioid, cocaine, and cannabis use disorders [25]. DSM-III-R and DSM-IV had good to excellent reliability in most items in opiates, cannabis, and cocaine [26]. Composite International Diagnostic Interview Substance Abuse Module (CIDI-SAM) is derived from another famous interview psychiatric instrument CICI. CIDI-SAM can be utilized to test alcohol, tobacco, and nine classes of psychoactive drug disorders. The performance of CIDI-SAM was excellent in most target substance in the reliability test [23].

Based on DSM series, some other drug dependence scales have been developed. Substance Dependence Severity Scale (SDSS) is to test drug dependences' mental disorders, based on DSM-IV and ICD (mental health tests), as well as drug use history, such as frequency, recency, and amount of consumption in last 30 days [24]. It has 11 items to assess the severity and frequency, scored from 0 to 49, and higher score means higher severity level. SDSS had excellent performance in most items in alcohol, cocaine, heroin, and sedatives in test-retest. Semi-structured Assessment for Drug Dependence and Alcoholism (SSADDA) and The Chemical, Use, Abuse, and Dependence Scale (CUAD) are also DSM-based instruments. SSADDA has seven criteria to test a large range of indexes, including drug use history, social activities, and physical and psychological problems. SSADDA performed excellent in nicotine and opioid dependence, good in alcohol and cocaine, and fair in cannabis, sedatives, and stimulants [27]. CUAD relies heavily on the American Psychiatric Association's (1987) Diagnostic and DSM-III-R for substance use disorders [28, 29]. CUAD has maximum 80 items and has Substance Severity Score for each substance they used and Total Severity Score for all substance they used. Different from assessments mentioned above, CUAD has different score weight for different items. For example, for items 16 and 17, each item scores 4 points, but 3 points for item 15, if they are true. In test-retest reliability, CUAD performed with excellence [29].

Evaluating the severity of withdrawal symptoms is as important as assessing the severity when patients are using drugs. There are a group of assessments focusing on the severity of opiate dependence in withdrawal. Severity of Opiate Dependence Questionnaire (SODQ) is a self-completion questionnaire that contains five sections for opiate dependence. It assesses opiate use, physical and affective symptoms in withdrawal, withdrawal-relief drug use, and rapidity of reinstatement of withdrawal symptoms after a period of abstinence. This assessment concerns more about the severity in withdrawal. The reliability was from 0.70 to 0.88 in Cronbach's alpha [30]. The Clinical Opiate Withdrawal Scale (COWS) is an 11-item clinician-administered instrument to assess opioid withdrawal severity [31]. COWS also has different score weights on different items. The possible maximum score is 48. The score represents the level of severity, 5–12 points: "mild," 13–24: "moderate," 25–36: "moderately severe," and more than 36: severe (more than 36, 33). The reliability of overall items in Cronbach's alpha is 0.78 [31]. There are several similar withdrawal scales focusing on opiates, such as The Himmelsbach Scale, The Opiate Withdrawal Scale, Subjective Opiate Withdrawal Scale, Objective Opiate Withdrawal Scale, Short Opiate Withdrawal Scale, and The Subjective Opiate Withdrawal Questionnaire [32–36]. Clinical Drug Use Scale (DUS) can assess the drug dependence severity in different stages. It is a self-report instrument with excellent reliability to scale abstinence, consumption without impairment, abuse, dependence, and dependence with institutionalization [37, 38].

Some instruments tend to use a large number of questions to obtain detailed information from drug dependences and some tend to use a small number of items to diagnose patients' severity as soon as possible. Similar to CUAD, 80 items, Substance Abuse Outcomes Module (SAOM) is a 113-item self-report scale. It covers patient characteristic, patient outcomes, and process of care. This assessment takes 20 minutes on average [39]. On the other hand, The Severity of Dependence Scale (SDS), Leeds Dependence Questionnaire (LDQ), SDSS, Drug use disorder (DUD), and COWS have much fewer items. SDS has five items to measure the level of drug dependence, mainly focusing on psychological components [40]. (LDQ) has 10 self-completion items, which are sensitive to severity change over time in opiate and alcohol dependences [41]. In both SDS and LDQ, each of the items can be scored from 0 to 3 and higher score represents higher level of drug dependence [40, 41]. DUD is a self-report measurement to assess drug use and dependence criteria for marijuana, cocaine, and painkiller. It tried to minimize the subjects' bias while designing [42]. The number of items does not represent the reliability. No matter large number items assessments, CUAD and SAOM or small number items SDS, LDQ, DUD, and COWS, both had good to excellent performance in reliability test, details in **Table 1**.

2.3 Treatment outcomes assessments

Evaluating drug use–related disorders during treatment is crucial and treatments can be according to this. The assessments mentioned in severity diagnosis assessments can also be utilized during treatment. However, here are some methods that have been designed for it. SAOM, The Substance Abuse Treatment Scale (SATS), Australian Treatment Outcomes Profile (ATOP), Treatment Outcomes Profile (TOP) are focusing on the treatment outcomes in drug dependences. SATS measures the treatment progress for drug dependences. SATS and TOP monitor and assess patients with eight scales and 38 items, respectively [43, 44]. TOP covers more fields including substance use, health risk behavior, offending, and health and social functioning. In reliability

Assessments	Target substance	Number of items	Approach	Reliability*
Screening assessments				
CAGE-AID	Drugs	4 sections[a]	Self-report	Generally good to excellent
Prenatal substance abuse screen (5Ps)	alcohol and drugs	5 items	self-report	not tested
The Alcohol, Smoking and Substance Involvement Screening Test (ASSIST)	alcohol, cigarettes and drugs	8 items	Self-report	0.58–0.90
The Drug Abuse Screening Test (DAST)	alcohol and drugs	28 items	Self-report	0.86–0.91 in Internal Consistency Reliability
Two-item conjoint screening (TICS)	alcohol and drugs, particularly sensitive to polysubstance	5 items	Semi-structured interview	Can screen nearly 80% drug dependences with disorders
Severity diagnoses assessments				
Addiction Severity Index (ASI)	Alcohol and drugs	Covering 7 problem areas	Semi-structured interview	Generally reliable, good to excellent
Clinical Drug Use Scale (DUS)	Drugs	5 sections	Self-report	Generally excellent
Composite International Diagnostic Interview Substance Abuse Module (CIDI-SAM)	Alcohol, tobacco and nine classes of psychoactive drugs		Fully-structured interview	Generally excellent
Drug Use Scale (DUS)	Drugs	5 items	Self-report	Generally excellent
DSM series	Drugs	—	Interviews	Most items were good to excellent in DSM-IV and 5
Leeds Dependence Questionnaire (LDQ)	Alcohol and opiates	10 items	Self-report	0.70–0.90
Semi-structured Assessment for Drug Dependence and Alcoholism (SSADDA)	Drugs, particular for cocaine and opioid	7 sections	Semi-structured interview	Excellent in cocaine and opioids, fair to good in other drugs, fair to good in psychiatric disorders
Severity of Opiate Dependence Questionnaire (SODQ)	Opiates	5 sections	Self-report	0.70–0.88 in Cronbach's alpha test
Substance Dependence Severity Scale (SDSS)	Alcohol and drugs	11 items	Semi-structured interview	Most items were excellent in alcohol, cocaine, heroin, and sedatives

Assessments	Target substance	Number of items	Approach	Reliability*
The Chemical, Use, Abuse, and Dependence Scale (CUAD)	Alcohol and drugs	Minimum 2 items, maximum 80 items	Semi-structured interview	Generally excellent
The Clinical Opiate Withdrawal Scale (COWS)	Buprenorphine, opiates and opioids	11 items	Self-report	0.78 in Cronbach's alpha
The Severity of Dependence Scale (SDS)	Drugs	5 items	Self-report	0.8–0.9 in Cronbach's alpha
The Substance Abuse Treatment Scale (SATS)	Drugs	8 scales	Semi-structured interview	Generally excellent
Treatment outcomes assessments				
Australian Treatment Outcomes Profile (ATOP)	Alcohol and drugs	22 items		Excellent in most items
Drug Use Disorder (DUD)	Marijuana, cocaine and painkillers	12 items	Self-report	0.88–0.95 in Cronbach's a coefficient
Drug Use Disorder (DUD)	Marijuana, cocaine and painkillers	12 items	Self-report	0.88–0.95 in Cronbach's a coefficient
Substance Abuse Outcomes Module (SAOM)	Alcohol and drugs	113 items	Self-report	Moderate to high
Treatment Outcomes Profile (TOP)	Drugs	38 items	Fully-structured interview	Eight items below 0.6 and eight more than 0.75
Objective severity scoring index (OSSI)	Narcotics	An equation	—	Not tested

**the reliability test is test-retest, if there is no indication; the coefficient is larger than 0.75, the reliability is excellent, 0.6–0.74 is good and 0.4–0.59 is fair.*
[a]one section might contain more than one item.

Table 1.
The list of screening and severity diagnosis assessments.

test [45], SAT had excellence in test-retest [43]. Eight items of TOP reached 0.75, and eight items are below 0.6 [45]. ATOP was proposed by Australia researchers to assess alcohol or drug use and its risk profile, general health, and well-being. ATOP contains 22 items and averagely scored more than 0.7 in test-retest [46]. In test-retest, ATOP had 19 items excellent, 1 item good, and 2 poor.

Zilm and Sellers (1978) proposed a quantitative technique to assess the level of physical dependence of narcotics, with administering naloxone [47]. They gave an equation of objective severity scoring index (OSSI). However, this method has not been tested in reliability or validity, and Zilm and Sellers claim it relies on the experience of executors.

2.4 Assessments selecting

All assessments are listed in **Table 1**. It concludes the target substance, number of questions, assessment approach, and reliability. The reliability is from test-retest, and the reliability coefficient below 0.40 is Poor; 0.40 to 0.59 is Fair, 0.60–0.74 is Good, and 0.75–1.00 is Excellent [48]. There are other assessments, such as Antisocial Personality Disorder, CIDI, General Health Questionnaire, Primary Care Posttraumatic Stress Disorder Screen, Health of the Nation Outcome Scales, and Michigan Alcoholism Screening Test, designed for psychological or alcoholic diagnosis and are not discussed in detail in this review.

Two main approaches of drug use disorder severity assessments are interview and self-report. In terms of reliability, there is no significant difference between interview and self-report. Several studies have proved that self-report assessments are as reliable as interview ones [49–51]. Compared with interview, self-report is more cost-effective and convenient, but the understanding of questions might affect the accuracy of self-report. Moreover, self-report instrument is more likely to collect honest answers and face-to-face interview might be unsuccessful to, because the questions would make the interviewees uncomfortable [52]. In interview assessments, there are two types, semi-structured and fully structured. Both of them have advantages and disadvantages. Fully structured interview does not need clinical judgment, and as a result, it does not need experienced clinicians. Semi-structured interview, in contrast, can obtain more detailed information of patients' status, but more human cost and time cost [53].

Specific to each instrument, the reliability has been listed above, and all assessments are generally reliable. Some studies compared different assessments and found no significant difference in general, but disagreement in specific field [54, 55]. For example, the reliabilities of SDSS for alcohol, cocaine, heroin, and sedatives were excellent, but for cannabis, it was just fair [24]. SSADDA is more sensitive to cocaine and opioid [27]. In addition, the validity of assessments may not vary between different races. Taking DSM-IV as an example, Horton et al. reported that there is no significant difference between African-Americans and Caucasians, when using this assessment [55]. Taken together, when screening instruments or severity assessments were selected, factors, including genders, different stages of drug use or withdrawal, reliability in different drugs, time, human resource and economic cost, and the condition of patients, should be considered. It is important to choose one or more assessments, based on patients' conditions to get accurate results.

3. Treatments

The treatments for drug dependence can be classified into three categories, conventional treatments (non-emergency), emergency (overdose) treatments, and novel treatments. Psychosocial interventions and medication managing are the most common techniques in conventional treatments. Patients need pharmacological intervention to reverse death when they are in overdose. In addition, physical activities, brain stimulation, virtual reality (VR), and mindfulness are considered as novel treatments for drug dependence. The drug dependences may need a combined treatment to make the therapeutic process more effective.

3.1 Conventional treatments

WHO and The United Nations Office on Drugs and Crime gave the standards of the treatments for drug use disorders (Standards). In order to screen out unqualified (ineffective, even harmful) treatments, Standards required the treatments of drug disorders to meet: (1) stopping or dropping drug use; (2) improving health, well-being, and social functioning of the affected individuals; (3) preventing future harms by reducing the risk of complications and relapse [4]. According to Standards, the traditional treatments can be categorized into psychosocial interventions, medication managing treatments and overdose or emergency treatments.

3.1.1 Psychosocial interventions

Psychosocial interventions are to address psychological and psychosocial issues related to drug use disorders. Cognitive-behavioral therapy (CBT) helps patients identify self-defeating thoughts and behaviors. It can contribute to address mental illnesses caused or related to drug use [4, 56]. Previous studies provided data-based evidence to support the effectiveness of CBT in drug dependence [57–59]. Contingency management (CM) is to reinforce patients' positive behaviors, such as keeping abstinence, treatment attendance, and compliance with medication, by providing them rewards. Different from other treatments, the effect of CM may be not directly shown in drug use reduction, but shown in combined treatments [4, 60].

Moreover, building connection with other individuals and obtaining supports from others are crucial in psychological therapy. Family-orientated treatment approaches (FOTAs) are to realize the importance of family relationships and cultures. FOTA has been proved that it can be an effective and promising method for drug use disorders [61]. Mutual-help groups (MHP) are frequently used in drug rehabilitation centers, and there are famous drug-focused mutual-help groups, such as Narcotics Anonymous and Cocaine Anonymous. Twelve-step oriented MHP is a nonprofessional, mental support, emphasizing "sharing" and peer-led treatment [4, 62]. Evidence from different types of studies, meta-analysis, randomized controlled trials, and observational studies illustrated the effects of MHP, including reducing drug use, improving mental health, and decreasing relapse rate [63–65]. There are also some other psychosocial interventions, such as contingency management, the community reinforcement approach, and motivational interviewing and motivational enhancement therapy.

3.1.2 Medication managing treatments

Medication managing, also called substitution therapy, is useful and effective in managing and treating drug-related disorders. Pharmacological techniques treat drug disorders, usually through agonist approaches, antagonist approaches, targeting negative reinforcement of drugs, and targeting psychiatric and cognitive disorders [66]. Different drugs have different targeted medicines. For opioid dependence, WHO suggests two main pharmacological treatments: (1) opioid agonist maintenance treatment with long-acting opioids (extended-release opioids), methadone and buprenorphine, this method should be combined with psychosocial treatments; (2) detoxification, with naltrexone, an opioid antagonist [67]. Some other synthetic oral opioids such as L-alpha-acetyl-methadol and slow-release morphine are also considered as effective agents for opioids withdrawal [68]. Long-acting benzodiazepine is a helpful medicine for sedative, hypnotic, or anxiolytic withdrawal. In addition, for methamphetamine and cocaine withdrawal, Provigil and immunotherapies would be the most useful agents, respectively [68–71]. These medicines will reduce withdrawal symptoms and reduce drug use, rather than being an alternative addiction for another [72].

3.1.3 Conventional treatments selecting

The conventional treatments do not have a specific program for patients in different levels of severity. Taking cocaine dependence as example, Hser et al. claim that different treatments, including outpatient methadone maintenance, outpatient drug-free, long-term residential and short-term inpatient, did not have significant difference on different severity of cocaine [73]. In general, a combined treatment is more effective. Drug-free treatments are more suitable for less severe drug dependence, and high level of drug dependence is challenge for any treatments.

Different groups may need different treatments. For pregnant women, almost all pharmacological treatments, except methadone, are unavailable, and stimulants and cannabis substitution drug is very limited, even nonexistent [74, 75]. Psychosocial intervention might be a better method [75]. Moreover, the treatments should be changed based on different ages. Treatment Improvement Protocol suggests that the elderly with drug addiction should accept age-specific treatments and combined pharmacological and psychosocial treatment is necessary. Building and rebuilding of self-esteem and social support network are important [76]. Adolescents with drug addiction may confront worse psychiatric comorbidity, and this issue is more common in family having alcohol and drug problems and mental health problems [77, 78]. Family dysfunction and mental health problems are more common and worse in girls, compared with boys [79, 80]. Therefore, the treatments for adolescents may focus more on psychiatric issues, and solving family issues would benefit the treatment outcomes, especially for female adolescents.

Treatments also need to consider about ethical issues. A large proportion of dependences are not willing to accept or seek treatments [45, 81]. Compulsory drug treatment is not legal in some nations, and how to convince drug dependences to receive treatments is a challenge. Johnson intervention, which is an organized and rehearsed meeting to let the drug dependence understand the treatment benefits and nontreatment risks, can be a choice [82]. In addition, patients should choose the treatments they prefer. For example, according to Drug Abuse Treatment Outcome Study, cocaine dependent did not like methadone maintenance. Patients who have used but are not dependent on heroin and cocaine like drug-free treatments more. Heroin dependence, or cocaine and heroin dependence, tends to be treated in methadone maintenance program [73].

3.2 Overdose or emergency treatments

Opioids and stimulants overdose can cause irreversible damage, even death. Opioid dependences are more likely to experience overdose, especially using it by injection [4]. WHO suggests that naloxone, a life-saving drug, can be timely administrated to reserve the opioid overdose [83]. For stimulants overdose, WHO recommends using benzodiazepines and sometimes antipsychotic medications to manage syndromes and ameliorate symptoms [4]. Gorelick claim that pharmacokinetic, which is to maintain the target drug under its minimum effective concentration at the site of action, treatment can be effective for acute drug overdose [84]. The immunotherapies are antagonizing the effects of drug through pharmacokinetic mechanisms. This approach involves the use of nicotine-specific antibodies that bind nicotine in serum, resulting in a decrease in nicotine distribution to the brain and an increase in nicotine's elimination half-life [85].

3.3 Novel treatments

Psychosocial and pharmacological interventions are treating drug disorders through reducing negative symptoms, decreasing craving, or managing the effect of target drugs. New treatment methods bring prospects for the cure of addiction, and it is helpful for developing personalized and comprehensive treatment.

Recent studies have highlighted the potential of brain stimulation as an innovative, safe, and cost-effective treatment for some SUDs. These include: (i) transcranial electrical stimulation; (ii) transcranial magnetic stimulation (TMS); (iii) transcranial direct current stimulation (tDCS); and (iv) deep brain stimulation (DBS). Stimulation therapies may achieve their effect through direct or indirect modulation of brain regions involved in addiction, either acutely or through plastic changes in neuronal transmission. Although these mechanisms are not well understood, further identification of the underlying neurobiology of addiction and rigorous evaluation of brain stimulation methods has the potential for unlocking an effective, long-term treatment of addiction.

Exercise may also provide a new treatment idea. In recent years, exercises are considered as a novel treatment for drug addiction. Lynch et al. concluded that exercises can reduce the reinforcing effects of drugs and may prevent the relapse [86]. Exercise can increase dopamine level in several parts of brain [87], bring happiness [88], and improve mental health and self-esteem [89]. More importantly, some studies found that exercises can affect dopamine in the reward pathway, even repair the decreased dopamine receptors [86, 90–92]. Furthermore, the side effects that resulted by drug use are not only psychiatric disorders and brain damage, but also the physical impairment, such as impaired respiratory system and bone loss [93, 94]. Exercise can benefit the physical health is well known. Drug dependences should accept the risk evaluation of exercise before having physical activities. The effects of exercises on drug use disorders still need more clinical studies, especially on the dopamine system. Besides, depending on the age, type of drug, age of onset, it is necessary to design appropriate exercise plans according to individual health characteristics [95]. It reported a significant increase in glutamate and GABA signaling in the visual cortex following exercise, as well as an increase in glutamate in the ACC after exercise in adult rats, and exercise-induced expansion of cortical pools can be seen for both glutamate and GABA neurons [96]. Additional, high-intensity interval training has been noted to possess benefits even greater than those of standard moderate exercise [97]. However, appropriate exercise intensity and exercise mode for patient with different age, gender, type of drug still need more in-depth research.

Besides, VR technology has emerged as a powerful tool for the research and intervention of addiction [98]. It's a tool to study how proximal multi-sensorial cues, contextual environmental cues, as well as their interaction (complex cues), modulate addictive behaviors. Moreover, VR simulations can be personalized. They are currently refined for psychotherapeutic interventions. Embodiment, eye-tracking, and neurobiological factors represent novel future directions. The progress of VR applications has bred auspicious ways to advance the understanding of treatment mechanisms underlying addictions.

Last but not least, mindfulness-based relapse prevention (MBRP) has been shown as effective in treating substance use disorders [99]. Study results suggest that mindfulness meditation practice may produce endogenous theta stimulation in the prefrontal cortex, thereby enhancing inhibitory control over opioid dose escalation behaviors [100]. However, it necessary to examine the following mediators of intervention outcome: mindfulness skills, emotion regulation skills, executive functioning skills, savoring, and positive and negative affect.

4. Conclusion and outlook

For more than 40 years, the instruments to assess the severity of drug dependence have been developed well, and different quantitative methods can cover almost every field of the symptoms in different periods and stages of drug addiction. Patients, medical workers, or researchers can choose suitable assessments, based on their conditions. The comprehensive and convenient techniques might leave one problem that is how to convince the dependences to do the screening or diagnosis tests. As mentioned in Treatments section, most drug dependences do not want to accept treatments. This needs efforts from drug dependences themselves, their family, the community, and whole society.

Drug addiction is a chronic disease [101], it needs chronic treatments. The interventions or treatments for drug dependence might be in a dilemma caused by medical development. Existing treatments are focusing on addressing the symptoms of drug use–related disorders, rather than the root of addiction. Drug addiction, also called drug use disorders, is defined as a complex, but treatable, disease that affects brain functions modulated by genetic, developmental, and environmental factors. People with addiction use drugs often tend to continue despite harmful consequences [101, 102]. The brain function damage caused by drug use has been proved. For example, chronic methamphetamine use can result in hippocampal volumes decrease and severe gray-matter deficits [103]. Moreover, dopamine receptors and transporters deficits are the consequence of drug use [104, 105]. Conventional treatments, psychosocial interventions, and medicines can only ameliorate withdrawal symptoms, reduce craving or improve psychological health, but not repair the brain or dopamine functions. Exercise or brain stimulation might be a supportive method to contribute to brain system recovering. So far, it is far more from the real rehabilitation. We need more novel treatments to contribute to the functional recovery. Furthermore, existing treatments do not subdivide patients of different level of severity or different groups of patients. Future work can design treatments based on the characteristics of the patients.

Funding

This work was supported by Anhui University Natural Science Research Project (No. KJ2020A1057), the major science and technology projects in Anhui Province (No. 202103a07020004).

Author details

Mu Wang[1†], Yu-Xiang Qian[2†], Zeng-Hui Ding[1*], Cun-Feng Yuan[3], Xian-Jun Yang [1], Yu Liu[4] and Yi-Ning Sun[1]

1 Institute of Intelligent Machines, HFIPS, Chinese Academy of Sciences, Hefei, Anhui, PR China

2 Anhui Vocational College of Police Officers, PR China

3 Bureau of Drug Rehabilitation Administration, Ministry of Justice of the People's Republic of China, PR China

4 Anhui Mental Health Center, PR China

*Address all correspondence to: dingzenghui@iim.ac.cn

† These authors contributed equally to this work.

References

[1] 2018 WDR. Executive Summary Conclusions and Policy Implications: The United Nations Office on Drugs and Crime. 2018. Available from: https://www.unodc.org/wdr2018/en/topics.html

[2] Statistics NCfH. Overdose Death Rates. 2021. Available from: https://www.drugabuse.gov/drug-topics/trends-statistics/overdose-death-rates

[3] Center NDI. National Drug Threat Assessment. Washington, DC: U.S.: Department of Justice; 2011

[4] World Health Organization, Crime UNOoD. International standards for the treatment of drug use disorders: Revised edition incorporating results of field-testing. Geneva: World Health Organization; 2020

[5] SAMHSA. Screening and Assessment of Co-Occurring Disorders in the Justice System. Rockville: HHS Publication; 2015

[6] Sharon D, Dingle Genevieve JLN. Screening and Assessment of Comorbidity. Interventions for Addictions: Comprehensive Addictive Behaviors and Disorders. Oxford, United Kingdom: Elsevier; 2013

[7] Group WAW. The Alcohol, Smoking and Substance Involvement Screening Test (ASSIST): Development, reliability and feasibility. Addiction. 2002;**97**(9):1183-1194

[8] Organization WH. The Alcohol, Smoking and Substance Involvement Screening Test (ASSIST). 2010

[9] Brown RL, Saunders LA, Papasouliotis O. A two-item conjoint screen for alcohol and other drug problems. Journal of American Board Family Practice. 2001;**14**(2):95-106

[10] Chasnoff IJ, Wells AM, McGourty RF, LK B. Validation of the 4P's Plus © screen for substance use in pregnancy validation of the 4P's Plus. Journal of Perinatology. 2007;**27**(12):744-748

[11] Skinner HA. The drug abuse screening test. Addictive Behaviors. 1982;**7**(4):363-371

[12] Yudko E, Lozhkina O, Fouts A. A comprehensive review of the psychometric properties of the Drug Abuse Screening Test. Journal of Substance Abuse Treatment. 2007;**32**(2):189-198

[13] Brown RL, Rounds LA. Conjoint screening questionnaires for alcohol and other drug abuse: Criterion validity in a primary care practice. Wisconsin Medical Journal. 1995;**94**(3):135-140

[14] Basu D, Ghosh A, Hazari N, Parakh P. Use of Family CAGE-AID questionnaire to screen the family members for diagnosis of substance dependence. Indian Journal of Medical Research. 2016;**143**(6):722-730

[15] Leonardson GR, Ness FK, Daniels MC, Kemper E, Koplin BA, Leonardson GA. Validity and reliability of the audit and cage-aid in northern plains American Indians. Psychological Reports. 2005;**97**(1):161-166

[16] McLellan AT, Luborsky L, Woody GE, O'Brien CP. An improved evaluation instrument for substance abuse patients: The addiction severity index. Journal of Nervous and Mental Diseases. 1980;**168**(1):26-33

[17] Hodgins DC, El-Guebaly N. More data on the Addiction Severity Index:

Reliability and validity with the mentally ill substance abuser. Journal of Nervous and Mental Disease. 1992;**180**(3):197-201

[18] McLellan AT, Luborsky L, Cacciola J, Griffith J, Evans F, Barr HL, et al. New data from the Addiction Severity Index: Reliability and validity in three centers. Journal of Nervous and Mental Disease. 1985;**173**(7):412-423

[19] Organization WH. Addiction Severity Index - Lite Version (ASI-Lite)

[20] Ljungvall H, Persson A, Åsenlöf P, Heilig M, Ekselius L. Reliability of the Addiction Severity Index self-report form (ASI-SR): A self-administered questionnaire based on the Addiction Severity Index composite score domains. Nordic Journal of Psychiatry. 2020;**74**(1):9-15

[21] Association AP. DSM History. Available from: https://www.psychiatry.org/psychiatrists/practice/dsm/history-of-the-dsm

[22] Houts AC. Fifty years of psychiatric nomenclature: Reflections on the 1943 War Department Technical Bulletin, Medical 203. Journal of Clinical Psychology. 2000;**56**(7):935-967

[23] Cottler LB, Robins LN, Helzer JE. The reliability of the CIDI-SAM: A comprehensive substance abuse interview. British Journal of Addiction. 1989;**84**(7):801-814

[24] Gloria M, Carpenter KM, Cockerham MS, Trautman KD, Blaine J, Hasin S. Substance Dependence Severity Scale (SDSS): Reliability and validity of a clinician-administered interview for DSM-IV substance use disorders. Drug and Alcohol Dependence. 2000;**59**(1):63-75

[25] Denis CM, Gelernter J, Hart AB, Kranzler HR. Inter-observer reliability of DSM-5 substance use disorders. Drug and Alcohol Dependence. 2015;**153**:229-235

[26] Easton C, Meza E, Mager D, Ulüg B, Kilic C, Göğüş A, et al. Test-retest reliability of the alcohol and drug use disorder sections of the schedules for clinical assessment in neuropsychiatry (SCAN). Drug and Alcohol Dependence. 1997;**47**(3):187-194

[27] Pierucci-Lagha A, Gelernter J, GraceChan AA, Cubells JF, Farrer L, et al. Reliability of DSM-IV diagnostic criteria using the semi-structured assessment for drug dependence and alcoholism (SSADDA). Drug and Alcohol Dependence. 2007;**91**(1):85-90

[28] Association AP. Diagnostic and statistical manual of mental disorders III Revised. AP, Washington, DC; 1987

[29] McGovern MP, DH M. The Chemical Use, Abuse, and Dependence Scale (CUAD). Rationale, reliability, and validity. Journal of Substances and Abuse Treatment. 1992;**9**(1):27-38

[30] Sutherland G, Edwards G, Taylor C, Phillips G, Gossop M, Brady R. The measurement of opiate dependence. British Journal of Addiction. 1986;**81**:485-494

[31] Andrew Tompkins D, Bigelow GE, Harrison JA, Johnson RE, Fudala PJ, Strain EC. Concurrent validation of the Clinical Opiate Withdrawal Scale (COWS) and single-item indices against the Clinical Institute Narcotic Assessment (CINA) opioid withdrawal instrument. Drug and Alcohol Dependence. 2009;**105**(1-2):154-159

[32] Wesson DR, Ling W. The Clinical Opiate Withdrawal Scale (COWS). Journal of Psychoactive Drugs. 2003;**35**(2):253-259

[33] Himmelsbach K. The morphine abstinence syndrome, its nature and treatment. Annals of Internal Medicine. 1941;**15**(5):829-839

[34] Bradley BP, Gossop M, Phillips GT, Legarda JJ. The Development of an Opiate Withdrawal Scale (OWS). British Journal of Addiction. 1987;**82**(10):1139-1142

[35] Gossop M. The development of a short opiate withdrawal scale (SOWS). Addictive Behaviors. 1990;**15**(5):487-490

[36] Loimer N, Linzmayer L, Grünberger J. Comparison between observer assessment and self rating of withdrawal distress during opiate detoxification. Drug and Alcohol Dependence. 1991;**28**(3):265-268

[37] Drake RE, Mueser K, McHugo GJ. Outcomes Assessment in Clinical Practice. Baltimore: Williams & Wilkins; 1996

[38] Møller T, Linaker OM. Using brief self-reports and clinician scales to screen for substance use disorders in psychotic patients. Nordic Journal of Psychiatry. 2009;**64**(2):130-135

[39] Richard Smith G, Burnam A, Mosley CL, Hollenberg JA, Mancino M, Grimes W. Reliability and validity of the substance abuse outcomes module. Psychiatric Services. 2006;**57**(10):1452-1460

[40] Gossop M, Darke S, Griffiths P, Hando J, Powis B, Hall W, et al. The Severity of Dependence Scale (SDS): Psychometric properties of the SDS in English and Australian samples of heroin, cocaine and amphetamine users. Addiction. 1995;**90**(5):607-614

[41] Raistrick D, Bradshaw J, Tober G, Weiner J, Allison J, Healey C. Development of the Leeds Dependence Questionnaire (LDQ): A questionnaire to measure alcohol and opiate dependence in the context of a treatment evaluation package. Addiction. 1994;**89**(5):563-572

[42] Michael Scherer C, Furr-Holden D, Voas RB. Drug use disorder (DUD) questionnaire: Scale development and validation. Evaluation Review. 2013;**37**(1):35-58

[43] Mchugo GJ, Drake RE, Burton HL, Ackerson T. A scale for assessing the stage of substance abuse treatment in persons with severe mental illness. Journal of Nervous & Mental Disease. 1996;**183**(12):762-767

[44] Marsden J, Farrell M, Bradbury C, Dale-Perera A, Eastwood B, Roxburgh M, et al. Development of the treatment outcomes profile. Addiction. 2008;**103**(9):1450-1460

[45] Health NSoDUa. Results from the 2008, National Survey on Drug Use and Health: National Findings 2008

[46] Deacon RM, Mammen K, Bruno R, Mills L, Dunlop A, Holmes J, et al. Assessing the concurrent validity, inter-rater reliability and test–re-test reliability of the Australian Treatment Outcomes Profile (ATOP) in alcohol and opioid treatment populations. Addiction. 2020;**116**(5):1245-1255

[47] Zilm DH, Sellers EM. The quantitative assessment of physical dependence on opiates[J]. Drug & Alcohol Dependence. 1978;**3**(6):419-428

[48] Joseph L, Levin B, Paik MC. Statistical Methods for Rates and Proportions. New York: John Wiley & Sons Inc; 1981

[49] Motiuk M, Motiuk L, Bonta J. A comparison between self-report and

interview-based inventories in offender classification. Criminal Justice and Behavior. 1992;**19**:143-159

[50] Stuart A, Pasco J, Jacka F, Brennan S, Berk M, Williams L. Comparison of self-report and structured clinical interview in the identification of depression. Comprehensive Psychiatry. 2013;**55**(4):866-869

[51] Lopes AD, Vilar Furtado R, Silva Cayii CL, Malfatti CA. Comparison of self-report and interview administration methods based on the Brazilian versions of the Western Ontario Rotator Cuff Index and Disabilities of the Arm, Shoulder and Hand Questionnaire in patients with rotator cuff disorders. Clinics (Sao Paulo). 2009;**64**(2):121-125

[52] Treatment CfSA. Substance Abuse Treatment: Addressing the Specific Needs of Women. Chapter 4: Screening and Assessment. 2009 Available from: https://www.ncbi.nlm.nih.gov/books/NBK83253/

[53] Samet S, Waxman R, Hatzenbuehler M, Hasin DS. Assessing addiction: Concepts and instruments. Addiction Science and Clinical Practices. 2007;**4**(1):19-31

[54] Compton WM, Cottler LB, Dorsey KB, Spitznagel EL, Mager DE. Comparing assessments of DSM-IV substance dependence disorders using CIDI-SAM and SCAN. Drug and Alcohol Dependence. 1996;**41**(3):179-187

[55] Horton J, Compton W, Cottler LB. Reliability of substance use disorder diagnoses among African–Americans and Caucasians. Drug and Alcohol Dependence. 2000;**57**(3):203-209

[56] Centers AA. Cognitive Behavioral Therapy Techniques and Addiction Treatment 2020. Available from: https://americanaddictioncenters.org/cognitive-behavioral-therapy?__cf_chl_jschl_tk__=570a44de24cf03e4a5da9209dc74df8097732668-1613747602-0-AW2aefpBoLgIvUV2ezPvTp56xm5mo-qTNkLOpoeP0vl9mYcPPjXVCwHRjZ6xls3lGhXCCqPI8daI0jdPZJi4DimZ5jlfZBT95FpjCKl_rSo163cW-PtGSWay1MrPwGAa8ZqE_UsbK0DqVk1hgY4Bc2cLQO7W8XeaJGzQ5nIm_JdS5b2ka7GR-xLrCQjQZcnnsT_tpr0PLiZjEnmJ36BJ6eyyVfOMmdRUMUEpDXGNCl2WRW1vTDWiihmAjBj21YJGVMyvUZuS--pGJpbLlg28CB0UsHMeAnfn_vWiRvM9Cs_Ypp066s7c-2A_Chif7gK5mhuJTywgLE0f66Q8n483CV81H5PtmllOwWvbuY16DvV5oCmpiGk0zN75hBU2avGSD5w55MnXPbFWnCImMG3ELRs

[57] Dutra L, Stathopoulou G, Basden SL, Leyro TM, Powers MB, Otto MW. A meta-analytic review of psychosocial interventions for substance use disorders. American Journal of Psychiatry. 2008;**165**(2):179-187

[58] Magill M, Ray LA. Cognitive-behavioral treatment with adult alcohol and illicit drug users: A meta-analysis of randomized controlled trials. Journal of Studies on Alcohol and Drugs. 2009;**70**(4):516-527

[59] Ladan Z, Mehdi B, Farkhondeh S, Ebrahim MS. Anger management in substance abuse based on cognitive behavioral therapy: An interventional study. BMC Psychiatry. 2017;**17**(1):375

[60] Prendergast M, Podus D, Finney J, Greenwell L, Roll J. Contingency management for treatment of substance use disorders: A meta-analysis. Addiction. 2006;**101**(11):1546-1560

[61] Stanton DM. Family treatment approaches to drug abuse problems: A review. Family Process. 1979;**18**(3):251-280

[62] Kelly JF, Yeterian JD. 4—Mutual-help groups. In: O'Donohue WT, Cummings NA, editors. Evidence-Based Adjunctive Treatments. San Diego: Academic Press; 2008. pp. 61-105

[63] Crits-Christoph P, Siqueland L, Blaine J, Frank A, Luborsky L, Onken LS, et al. Psychosocial treatments for cocaine dependence: National Institute on Drug Abuse Collaborative Cocaine Treatment Study. Archives of General Psychiatry. 1999;**56**(6):493-502

[64] Weiss RD, Griffin ML, Gallop RJ, Najavits LM, Frank A, Crits-Christoph P, et al. The effect of 12-step self-help group attendance and participation on drug use outcomes among cocaine-dependent patients. Drug and Alcohol Dependence. 2005;**77**(2):177-184

[65] Fiorentine R, Hilhouse MP. Drug treatment and 12-step program participation: The additive effects of integrated recovery activities. Journal of Substance Abuse Treatment. 2000;**18**(1):65-74

[66] Potenza MN, Sofuoglu M, Carroll KM, Rounsaville BJ. Neuroscience of behavioral and pharmacological treatments for addictions. Neuron. 2011;**69**(4):695-712

[67] Organization WH. Guidelines for the psychosocially assisted pharmacological treatment of opioid dependence. 2009. Available from: https://www.who.int/publications/i/item/9789241547543

[68] Organization WH. Neuroscience of psychoactive substance use and dependence. 2004. Available from: https://www.who.int/substance_abuse/publications/en/Neuroscience.pdf

[69] Kinsey BM, Kosten TR. Active immunotherapy for the treatment of cocaine dependence. Drugs Future. 2010;**35**(4):301-306

[70] Karila L, Weinstein A, Aubin HJ, Benyamina A, Reynaud M, Batki SL. Pharmacological approaches to methamphetamine dependence: A focused review. Brithish Journal of Clinical Pharmacology. 2010;**69**(6):578-592

[71] Orson FM, Kinsey BM, Singh RAK, Wu Y, Gardner T, Kosten TR. Substance abuse vaccines. Annals of the New York Academy Science. 2008;**1141**:257-269

[72] Association AP. Opioid Use Disorder. 2018. Available from: https://www.psychiatry.org/patients-families/addiction/opioid-use-disorder/opioid-use-disorder

[73] Hser YI, Anglin MD, Fletcher B. Comparative treatment effectiveness: Effects of program modality and client drug dependence history on drug use reduction. Journal of Substance Abuse Treatment. 1998;**15**(6):513-523

[74] Rayburn WF, Bogenschutz MP. Pharmacotherapy for pregnant women with addictions. American Journal of Obstetrics and Gynecology. 2004;**191**(6):1885-1897

[75] Saia KA, Schiff D, Wachman EM, Mehta P, Vilkins A, Sia M, et al. Caring for pregnant women with opioid use disorder in the USA: Expanding and improving treatment. Current Obstetrics and Gynecology Reports. 2016;**5**(3):257-263

[76] F B. TIP 26: Substance Abuse Among Older Adults: Treatment Improvement Protocol (TIP) Series 26 1998. Available from: http://adaiclearinghouse.net/downloads/TIP-26-Substance-Abuse-Among-Older-Adults-67.pdf

[77] Rowe CL, Liddle HA, Greenbaum PE, Henderson CE. Impact of psychiatric comorbidity on treatment of adolescent drug abusers. Journal of Substance Abuse Treatment. 2004;**26**(2):129-140

[78] Grella CE, Hser Y-I, Joshi V. Drug treatment outcomes for adolescents with comorbid mental and substance use disorders. The Journal of Nervous and Mental Disease. 2001;**189**(6)

[79] Dakof GA. Understanding gender differences in adolescent drug abuse: Issues of comorbidity and family functioning. Journal of Psychoactive Drugs. 2000;**32**(1):25-32

[80] Rao UMA, Daley SE, Hammen C. Relationship between depression and substance use disorders in adolescent women during the transition to adulthood. Journal of the American Academy of Child & Adolescent Psychiatry. 2000;**39**(2):215-222

[81] MakarenkoI,MazhnayaA,PolonskyM, Marcus R, Bojko MJ, Filippovych S, et al. Determinants of willingness to enroll in opioid agonist treatment among opioid dependent people who inject drugs in Ukraine. Drug and Alcohol Dependence. 2016;**165**:213-220

[82] Johnson V. Intervention: How to Help Someone Who Doesn' t Want Help. MN, USA: Johnson Institute; 1986

[83] Organization WH. Opioid overdose. 2020. Available from: https://www.who.int/news-room/fact-sheets/detail/opioid-overdose

[84] Gorelick DA. Pharmacokinetic strategies for treatment of drug overdose and addiction. Future Medicine Chemistry. 2012;**4**(2):227-243

[85] LeSage MG, Keyler DE, Pentel PR. Current status of immunologic approaches to treating tobacco dependence: Vaccines and nicotine-specific antibodies. The AAPS Journal. 2006;**8**(1):E65-E75

[86] Lynch WJ, Peterson AB, Sanchez V, Abel J, Smith MA. Exercise as a novel treatment for drug addiction: A neurobiological and stage-dependent hypothesis. Neuroscience & Biobehavioral Reviews. 2013;**37**(8):1622-1644

[87] Foley TE, Fleshner M. Neuroplasticity of dopamine circuits after exercise: Implications for central fatigue. Neuromolecular Medicine. 2008;**10**(2):67-80

[88] Zhang Z-J, Chen W-Y. A systematic review of the relationship between physical activity and happiness. Journal of Happiness Studies. 2019;**20**

[89] Matta Mello Portugal E, Cevada T, Sobral Monteiro-Junior R, Teixeira Guimarães T, da Cruz RE, Lattari E, et al. Neuroscience of exercise: From neurobiology mechanisms to mental health. Neuropsychobiology. 2013;**68**(1):1-14

[90] Greenwood BN, Foley TE, Le TV, Strong PV, Loughridge AB, Day HEW, et al. Long-term voluntary wheel running is rewarding and produces plasticity in the mesolimbic reward pathway. Behavioural Brain Research. 2011;**217**(2):354-362

[91] Robison LS, Swenson S, Hamilton J, Thanos PK. Exercise reduces dopamine D1R and increases D2R in rats: Implications for addiction. Medical Science Sports and Exercise. 2018;**50**(8):1596-1602

[92] Robertson CL, Ishibashi K, Chudzynski J, Mooney LJ, Rawson RA, Dolezal BA, et al. Effect of exercise training on striatal dopamine D2/

D3 receptors in methamphetamine users during behavioral treatment. Neuropsychopharmacology. 2016;**41**(6):1629-1636

[93] Tashkin DP. Airway effects of marijuana, cocaine, and other inhaled illicit agents. Current Opinion in Pulmonary Medicine. 2001;7(2)

[94] Ding Z-H, Chen Y-Y, Wang X, Zhou X, Xu Y, Ma Z-C, et al. A comparison of bone quality and its determinants in young opioid-dependent women with healthy control group. Drug and Alcohol Dependence. 2017;**175**:232-236

[95] Ding ZH, Ma ZC, Yang XJ, Sun YN. Effect of eight-month exercise intervention on bone outcomes of young opioid-dependent women. International Journal of Environmental Research and Public Health. 2021;**18**(21)

[96] Rahman N, Mihalkovic A, Geary O, Haffey R, Hamilton J, Thanos PK. Chronic aerobic exercise: Autoradiographic assessment of GABA(a) and muopioid receptor binding in adult rats. Pharmacology and Biochemical. 2020;**196**

[97] Richard M, Gretchen C, Dione F, et al. Acute modulation of cortical glutamate and GABA content by physical activity. Journal of Neuroscience the Official Journal of the Society for Neuroscience. 2016

[98] Mazza M, Kammler-Sucker K, Lemenager T, Kiefer F, Lenz B. Virtual reality: A powerful technology to provide novel insight into treatment mechanisms of addiction. Translational Psychiatry. 2021;**11**(1)

[99] Hudak J, Hanley AW, Marchand WR, Nakamura Y, Yabko B, Garland EL. Correction: Endogenous theta stimulation during meditation predicts reduced opioid dosing following treatment with Mindfulness Oriented Recovery Enhancement. Neuropsychopharmacology. 2021;**46**(8):1544

[100] Hz A, Lu SB, Lr B, Lc C, Sl B, Lz D, et al. Study protocol for a randomized controlled trial of mindfulness-based relapse prevention for opioid use disorders. Contemporary and Clinical Trials. 2020;**99**

[101] Medicine ASoA. Definition of Addiction. 2019. Available from: https://www.asam.org/Quality-Science/definition-of-addiction

[102] Association AP. What Is a Substance Use Disorder? 2020

[103] Thompson PM, Hayashi KM, Simon SL, Geaga JA, Hong MS, Sui Y, et al. Structural abnormalities in the brains of human subjects who use methamphetamine. Journal of Neuroscience. 2004;**24**(26):6028-6036

[104] Gupta S, Kulhara P. Cellular and molecular mechanisms of drug dependence: An overview and update. Indian Journal of Psychiatry. 2007;**49**(2):85-90

[105] McCann UD, Kuwabar H, Kumar A, Palermo M, Abbey R, Brasic J, et al. Persistent cognitive and dopamine transporter deficits in abstinent methamphetamine users. Synapse. 2008;**62**(2):91-100

Chapter 4

Pattern of Substance Abuse among Children in Slum Areas of India

Sandeep Sitaram Kadu

Abstract

Background: We have been facing a frightening rise of substance abuse among the youngsters in recent years. Further, the problem is seen across all socioeconomic groups, from urban areas to small towns. However new substances are being abused which have also been documented. Substance abuse primarily among youth has been a matter of concern throughout the world. Study Design: It's a descriptive cross sectional study, done in collaboration with NGO (Balbhavan Project) working in slum areas of Ahmednagar. Duration of Study: 6 months. Material and Methods: Considering the time frame for the study, Research was carried out with the help of NGO working in slum areas of Ahmednagar and children fulfilling the inclusion and exclusion criteria. Data was collected with the help of predesigned questionnaire. It was estimated that the total sample size will be about 246 children who are using substances. (Calculated by open Epi Software).Results: The Result obtained at the end of our study was quite shocking. It was found that in slum area 87% children were drug abusers, among which 83% were boys and 17% were girls. A high correlation of substance abuse was found with increasing age. Most abused substance among them was Tobacco, Alcohol, Inhalants, Sedative and opium.

Keywords: substance abuse, tobacco, craving, slum area, children etc.

1. Introduction

Substance abuse is a social problem from eternity.World Health Organization (WHO) mentions substance abuse as the harmful or hazardous use of psychoactive substances, such as alcohol and illegal drugs. Substance abuse is "persistent or sporadic drug use inconsistent with or unrelated to acceptable medical practice" [1]. Substance abuse among the youngsters and adolescents is the rising social problem all over world [2].

Alcohol addiction is the leading problem for death and disability all over the world.it is observed that 75 million people are alcohol addicts and 3 million are opioid abusers in India [3]. Due to tobacco addiction nearly 13,000 deaths per day occurs all over It has been predicted by the According to World Health Organization (WHO) that tobacco consumption will lead more than 500 million mortality people by 2030 and it will be the commonest cause of death [4, 5]. Many studies has shown that smokers became habituated at adolescent period. It is unfortunate that consumption of alcohol is getting social acceptance and has become status symbol.

All hard drugs like opioids and other became the easily available which is the important cause of substance abuse in adolescents. Alcohol and opioid addiction is common in children. According to National institute on drug abuse (NIDA), in adolescence marijuana use consumption is common. Many studies had shown that common age group of substance abuse ranges from 12 to 20 years [6].

The United Nations has designed 17 Sustainable Development Goals (SDGs) and 169 targets. They expected that by 2030 all states will succeed to achieve all goals. From above all Sustainable Development Goals, important Goal-3 having Target-5 stresses on Strengthening the prevention of substance abuse and its proper treatment especially of narcotic drug and alcohol abuse. Many researches has confirmed that antisocial activities in childhood leads to alcohol abuse in adolescent. Adolescents is the most important stage of human life but unfortunately this group is most misunderstood and neglected by the society [7].

Substance addiction (drug addiction) and Non-substance addiction (behavioral addiction) are two different disorders. Substance addiction or drug addiction is a neuropsychiatric disorder categorized by a periodic craving for the consumption drug despite of having knowledge about harmful effects. Non substance abuse includes pathological food obsession, internet craving, and mobile phone compulsion [8].

Men are always under stress and for relief of it used many parameters one of it is drug abuse. This problem has risen at all levels in the society in various forms. Drug trafficking is one of the most profitable trades along with petroleum and weapons trade. Every country has and is facing this problem in its own way. Newer forms of drug abuse patterns like solvents are on the rise probably due to strict regulations on other recognized forms of abuse.

Street children in India constitute a group of marginalized population in most urban centers of the country. They constitute children living in streets permanently, who are detached from their families and live on the streets temporarily, children who belong to poor families and spend most of their time on the streets, children living with their families on the streets etc [9].

These children have to put up with a variety of physical and mental abuse and hence are a concern for a wide range of social issues. Poly substance abuse is common among these children and often solvents are the first psychoactive substance they attempt to try. Not much is known as to why children adopt such abusive behavior. Solvents are freely available in the market without any regulations in India. Though a lot of global awareness is reached about this form of abuse it is yet to be recognized by the political circle in the country [10].

We have been facing a shocking rise of substance abuse among the youngsters. Recent times have witnessed a steady increase in drug abuse among younger population, with more children starting substance use from an early age. Further, the delinquent is seen across all socioeconomic groups, from cities to small towns and rural areas, with new and multiple substance use also being recognized [11, 12].

Speedy industrial development with changing lifestyles have left the youth harassed for their survival; compelling many to seek defense in the dark world of substance abuse. India too, is fronting a similar condition that has been paying attention of policy makers and researchers [13–15].

Not only the child, but the family and society as a whole are likely to be disturbed as a result of early onset substance use. Thus, this matter is of nationwide interest and significance. This phase of life is characterized by growth and maturation of brain and body, which potentially affects responses to drugs and treatment [16–19].

World Health Organization (WHO) estimates that globally 25 to 90% of children and adolescents have consumed at least one substance of abuse [1, 19, 20]. In India approximately 5500 children and adolescents start using tobacco products daily, some as young as 10 years old. A large number of them have used tobacco prior to the age of 18 years [21–23].

Dependence is defined by World Health Organization and American Psychiatric Association, as a syndrome of physiological, behavioral and cognitive phenomena, which lead to loss of control over use. DSM-5, cancels the term 'dependence 'and substitutes it with 'use disorder' [24].

Research on substance abuse among children and adolescents presents its own distinctive challenges. But the main question is that why the Indian society is facing such a quandary where more of the teenagers and youths are indulging in immoral and unproductive activities like substance abuse. The present study has the aim of analyzing the biosocial profile and pattern of substance abusers. The study is indicative for the need of fostering a supportive environment comprising of both parents and teachers so that adolescents can adopt and sustain with the right choices for a healthy life.

1.1 Aims and objective

1. To assess the pattern and prevalence of substance abuse among Children in slum areas of Ahmednagar.

2. To find out demographic profile of children using substances for abuse.

3. To find out association of family history, peer pressure, educational status of family and children associated with substance use among children.

2. Methodology

It's a descriptive cross sectional study done in collaboration with NGO (Balbhavan Project) working in slum areas of Ahmednagar. They were evaluated according to pre designed questionnaire in given time frame with the help of NGO (Balbhavan project) working in that area. All the children satisfying the following inclusion and exclusion criteria were enrolled in the study.

2.1 Inclusion criteria

1. Children with age group 18 years or less of either sex were included in study.

2. Children who were willing to participate in research work.

3. Patients/Parent/relative/NGO who were ready to give informed consent.

4. Informed written consent was taken from the child or adolescent and the parent or NGO staff counselor (as a surrogate guardian, in case the parents are not available).

2.2 Exclusion criteria

1. Children with age group below 5 and above 18 years of either sex were not included.

2. A child who was Unable to provide information was not included in the study.

2.3 Sampling

For this research project we have chosen the most active non-governmental agency (NGO) of Ahmednagar, Maharashtra.This NGO named Snehalaya is working for the overall growth of children living in slum areas. They are also actively working on hot issue of substance abuse among these children. NGO has established nice rapport with children and also have data of the substance abuse among children. They also have information about the substance abuse and treatment of each child abuser. With help Snehalaya, we collected information related to our research project.

2.4 Sample size

Considering the time frame of the research, study was carried out with the help of NGO working in slum areas of Ahmednagar and children fulfilling the inclusion and exclusion criteria which were mentioned above. It was estimated that the total sample size will be about 246 children who are using substances. (Calculated by open Epi Software).

2.5 Working definition substance

The abusers are taking all kinds of substances commonly tobacco consumption, Bidi/Cigarette smoking, pan masala, gutkha, ganja, bhang, alcohol, LSD, Cocaine and Opium etc.

2.6 Substance abuser

We have labeled child as substance abuser who have fulfilled following criteria.

1-taking one or more above mentioned substances and consuming it since last 1 year,

2-using it at least once in a week or many times in last months.

2.7 Statistical analysis

Collected informations was tabulated and evaluated using suitable statistical tests as and when required. The information so collected was analyzed by using SPSS software. Chi-square test was used as per the requirement.

2.8 Results

To know the present scenario of substance abuse, we conducted a descriptive cross sectional study, among 246 children of slum areas of Ahmednagar under the guidance of Snehalay balbhavan project. The result obtained at the end of the study was quit shocking. It was found that in slum areas 87% children were drug abusers, among which 83% were boys and 17% were girls. A high correlation of substance abuse was found with increasing age consisting of 6.1% drug abuser of age group 5–8 years, 15% drug abuser of age group 9–12 years and 78.9% drug abuser of age group 13–18 years. Most abused substance among them was Tobacco, Alcohol, Inhalants, Sedative and opium. When we inquired about the educational status of parents, it was found that 84.6% of mothers were illiterate and 60.2% of fathers were illiterate. A special emphasis was laid on education of children among which 52% were school going and remaining were engaged in unskilled labor like rag picking, hotel worker, street vending, dhabha and other work. About 77.6% of these children got addicted due to their friends and 17.3% from their family. At the end of our study only 46.3% of them were willing to quit. 50.9% of children were craving for the substances and 38.8% of children got addicted due to peer pressure (**Tables 1-5** and **Figures 1** and **2**).

Sr. No.	Variable	Groups	No. of participants (N = 246)	Percentage (%)
1	Sex	Male	191	77.6
		Female	55	22.4
2	Age	5–8 years	15	6.1
		9–12 years	37	15.0
		13–18 years	194	78.9
3	Living arrangement	Home (With family)	191	77.6
		(with friends/ distant relatives)	55	22.4
4	Mothers literacy	Literate	38	15.4
		Illiterate	208	84.6
5	Fathers literacy	Literate	98	39.8
		Illiterate	148	60.2
6	Drug abuse by mother	Yes	197	80.1
		No	49	19.9
7	Drug abuse by father	Yes	207	84.1
		No	39	15.9
8	Work	Student	128	52.0
		Rag picker/ Kabadi	29	11.8
		Street level vending	9	3.7
		Dhaba/ Restaurant/ Waiter	5	2.0
		Unskilled worker/ Labourer	13	5.3
		Do not work	30	12.1
		Others	32	13.0

Table 1.
Demographic profile of participants.

Age Groups	Drug Abuse (%)	No Drug abuse (%)	Total	Chi-Square Value	P Value
5–8 years	6 (2.8)	9 (28.1)	15 (6.1)	41.517	0.000
9–12 years	27 (12.6)	10 (31.2)	37 (15.0)		
13–18 years	181 (84.6)	13 (40.6)	194 (78.9)		
Total	214 (100.0)	32 (100.0)	246 (100.0)		

As $p < 0.05$, there is significant association between age and drug abuse. Children in the age of 13–18 years are more likely to get involved in drug abuse.

Table 2.
Association between age and drug abuse.

Drug abuse by mother	Drug Abuse by children (%)	No Drug abuse by children (%)	Total	Chi-Square Value	P Value
Yes	178 (90.4)	19 (9.6)	197 (100.0)	9.887	0.004
No	36 (73.5)	13 (26.5)	49 (100.0)		
Total	214 (87.0)	32 (13.0)	246 (100.0)		

As $p < 0.05$, there is significant association between mother involved in drug abuse and drug abuse by the children. If the mother is using drugs, there are 90.4% chances of children getting involved in drug abuse.

Table 3.
Association between mothers involved in drug abuse and drug abuse by the children.

Drug abuse by father	Drug Abuse by children (%)	No Drug abuse by children (%)	Total	Chi-Square Value	P Value
Yes	188 (90.8)	19 (9.2)	207 (100.0)	16.920	0.000
No	26 (66.7)	13 (33.3)	39 (100.0)		
Total	214 (87.0)	32 (13.0)	246 (100.0)		

As $p < 0.05$, there is significant association between father involved in drug abuse and drug abuse by the children. If the father is using drugs, there are 90.8% chances of children getting involved in drug abuse.

Table 4.
Association between fathers involved in drug abuse and drug abuse by the children.

3. Discussion

Substance abuse refers to the harmful or hazardous use of psychoactive substance including alcohol and illicit drugs. The present study reveals the prevalence of substance abuse among children to be 87%, which is higher than that reported by Lisa Sarangi et al. [2] where the prevalence was 43.4%.Jasani PK et al.in his study covered 600 adolescents and he found that substance abusers children were 30.17% [25]. Another study conducted at Andhra Pradesh by Benegal et al. Prashant et al. [11] revealed that about 32.7% children were abusers. Many research studies have found that, in India 50% children up to grade nine experiences the substance at least once [26, 27].

This research study revealed the major basic reason behind such high consumption of substance abuse is poverty, easy availability of substances and peer pressure. Jasani PK et al. found that most common cause of substance abuse was peer pressure, then

Sr. No.	Variable	Groups	No. of participants (N = 246)	Percentage (%)
1	Substance abuse (N = 246)	Tobacco	140	56.9
		Alcohol	41	16.7
		Inhalant	23	9.3
		Sedative	6	2.4
		Opium	4	1.6
		No Substance abuse	32	13.0
2	Want to quit the habit (N = 214)	Yes	99	46.3
		No	115	53.7
3	Procurement of the drug (N = 214)	Friends	166	77.6
		Family	37	17.3
		Itself	11	5.1
4	Difficulty in quitting (N = 214)	Craving	109	50.9
		Peer pressure	83	38.8
		Easily available	17	7.9
		Withdrawal symptoms	5	2.4

Table 5.
Drug abuse & related parameters.

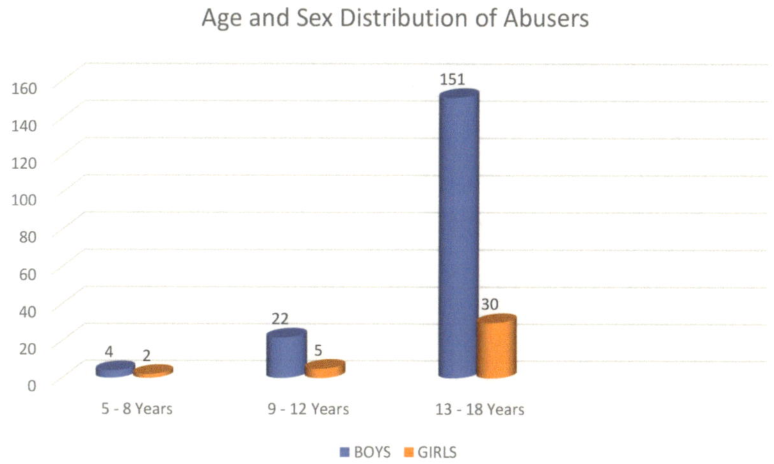

Figure 1.
Sex distribution among abusers.

experiencing thrill in life and academic stress [25]. Our results coincides with Benegal et al. Prashant et al. [11], in their study, they revealed most common reason was peer pressure (52.9%) then for pleasure (21.1%).But according to Jain et al. curiosity (68%) was the main reason for start of substance abuse [22], the reason behind it may be due to different culture and economic status. Another study by Barua et al. shown that

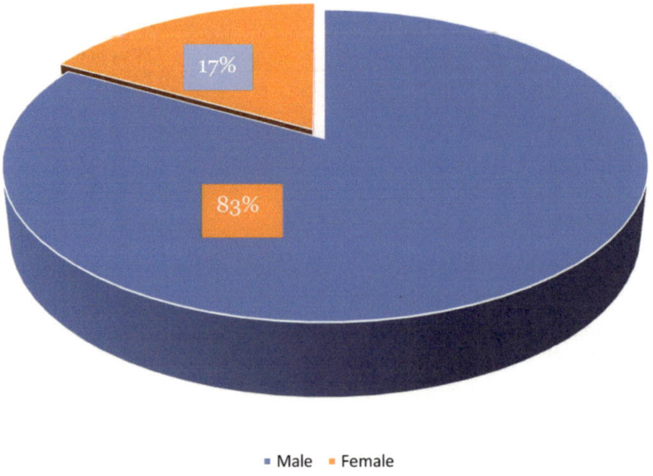

Figure 2.
Age and sex distribution of abusers.

academic stress comforting outcome and only for enjoyment were the common causes of consumption of alcohol [23].

This study also revealed that the most common substance being abused is the widely available Tobacco (56.9%) which is supporting, the findings of Dhirendra N. Sinha et al. [28]. Our findings are similar with Jasani PK et al., it showed most common substance is tobacco 25.83%, followed by liquor (2.17%), opioid/afin (1%) bhang (0.67%) [25].

Bihar based study by Sinha et al. showed that smoking is commonest substance abuse (19.4%)in school going children [14]. Kaur et al. from North India revealed 39.2% substance abusers consumes tobacco [15]. Another study from Uttar Pradesh by Dube and Handa et al. stated that alcohol is consumed by 22.8% abusers [16]. Similar findings 18.55% abusers are taking alcohol are also reported by Thacore [17], Shukla et al. described that 38.3% is substance abuse prevalence in the rural population in Uttar Pradesh [18]. Jena et al. also reported 28.8% rural people of Bihar consumes alcohol/drug [19]. Study conducted in most sensitive state, Punjab by Varma et al. revealed that 45.9% alcohol taking habit in urban population and 28.1% in rural population [20, 21].

It was found that in slum areas 87% children were drug abusers, among which 83% were boys and 17% were girls Prevalence of tobacco use was higher among boys than girls. Many research studies have found that, in India 50% children up to grade nine experiences the substance at least once [26, 27, 29]. Study by Majra et al. found that tobacco consumption is more among males (42.1%) as compared to females (17.0%) [13]. As boys are involved more in outdoor activities and are subjected to substance abuse. Adolescents reported using tobacco in multiple forms, chewing tobacco being the most popular.

A WHO study group on youth and drugs indicated that most of the experimentation and initiation of dependence producing drugs takes place during adolescence [30]. Though they had some knowledge about the harmful effects of substances, this was not sufficient to motivate them to quit, in our study only 46.3% were willing to quit. Craving (50.9%) was the most common cause to abstain substance abuse.

11 DSM-5 criteria implementation in clinics research purpose is easier than 11 DSM-IV criteria because one disorder is involved instead of two hierarchical disorders. A checklist helps for covering all criteria [31].

4. Conclusion

The study has emphasized the escalating incidence of substance abuse among slum children in Ahmednagar, pressing need of initiating programs for prevention and treatment in slum areas. The subject needs to be dealt in a comprehensive manner. There is need for availability of specialized treatment services for children who are using substances. These facilities should be available in government hospitals. The settings in which the facilities are delivered should be child sensitive and safe. Treatment programs must attempt to include the family in treatment and address the family issues as a part of the remedy. Rehabilitation of children should focus on skill building and vocational training. Substance abuse by children has detrimental impact on their physical, psychological, social and mental well-being hence needs immediate intervention. Rehabilitation of children abusing illicit substances is the necessity of the hour.

Acknowledgements

Firstly, I would like to express my sincere gratitude to my advisor Dr. Girish Kulkarni (Founder of Snehalaya) and Dr. Hanif for their great support. I am also thankful to all my students for their active participation in the project-Chhajed Neel A., Mehta Rahul J., Arve Rutvik N., Upadhyay Prabhakar I., Mustafa Saad.

Source of funding

Not applicable.

Conflict of interest

The author declares no conflict of interest in the present study.

Ethical clearance

Taken from institutional ethical committee.

Author details

Sandeep Sitaram Kadu
Department of Forensic Medicine, Dr. Vithalrao Vikhe Patil Foundation's Medical College, Ahmednagar, Maharashtra, India

*Address all correspondence to: dr.sandeepkadu@gmail.com

References

[1] WHO. Lexicon of Alcohol and Drug Terms. Geneva: world health organization; 1994

[2] Sarangi L, Acharya HP, Om PP. Substance abuse among adolescents in urban slums of Sambalpur. Indian Journal of Community Medicine. 2008;**33**(4):265-267

[3] Srivastava A, Pal H, Dwivedi SN, Pandey. A National Household Survey of drug abuse in India. In: Report Submitted to Ministry of Social Justice and Empowerment, Government of India and United Nations Office on Drugs and Crime. Regional Office for South Asia. Shastri Bhavan, New Delhi: Ministry of Social Justice and Empowerment, Government of India; 2002

[4] World Health Organization. Building Blocks for Tobacco Control, a Handbook. Geneva: World Health Organization; 2004. pp. 4-13

[5] Gupta PC, Sinha DN. Tobacco research in India. Indian Journal of Public Health. 2004;**48**(3):103-104

[6] Saddichha S, Manjunatha N, Khess CJ. Clinical course of development of alcohol and opioid dependence: What are the implications in prevention? Indian Journal of Community Medicine. 2010;**35**:359-361

[7] World Health Organization. Health Topics; Sustainable Development Goals (SDGs). www.who.int

[8] Zou Z, Wang H, d'Oleire Uquillas F, Wang X, Ding J, Chen H. Definition of substance and non-substance addiction. Advances in Experimental Medicine and Biology. 2017;**1010**:21-41. DOI: 10.1007/978-981-10-5562-1_2

[9] Kokiwar PR, Jogdand GR. Prevalence of substance use among male adolescents in an urban slum area of Karimnagar District, Andhra Pradesh. Indian Journal of Public Health. 2011;**55**(1):42-45

[10] Sharma R, Grover VL, Chaturvedi S. Tobacco use among adolescent students and the influence of role models. Indian Journal of Community Medicine. 2010;**35**(2):272-275

[11] Benegal V, Kulbhusan, Seshadri S, Karott M. Drug abuse among street children in Bangalore. A project in collaboration between NIMHANS, Bangalore and the Bangalore forum for street and working children, Monograph funded by CRY. 1998

[12] Ramachandran V. The prevention of alcohol related problems. Indian Journal of Psychiatry. 1991;**33**:3-10

[13] Majra JP, Basnet J. Prevalence of tobacco use among the children in the age group of 13-15 years in Sikkim after 5 years of prohibitory legislation. Indian Journal of Community Medicine. 2008;**33**(2):124-126

[14] Sinha DN. Tobacco and non-communicable disease. Indian Journal of Public Health. 2004;**48**:111-115

[15] Kaur J, Kishore J, Kumar M. Effect of anti-tobacco audiovisual messages on knowledge and attitude towards tobacco use in North India. Indian Journal of Community Medicine. 2012;**37**(4):227-231

[16] Dube KC, Handa SK. Drug use in health and mental illness in an Indian population. British Journal of Psychiatry. 1971;**118**:345-346

[17] Thacore VR. Drug abuse in India with special reference to Lucknow. Indian Journal of Psychiatry. 1972;**14**:257-261

[18] Shukla BR. Drinks and Drugs in a North Indian Village-an Anthropological Study. Lucknow, India: Ethnographic and Folk culture Society; 1979

[19] Jena R, Shukla TR, Hemraj P. Drug abuse in a rural community in Bihar: Some psychosocial correlates. Indian Journal of Psychiatry. 1996;**38**:43-46

[20] Varma VK, Singh A, Singh S, Malhotra AK. Extent and pattern of alcohol use in North India. Indian Journal of Psychiatry. 1980;**22**:331-337

[21] Lal B, Singh G. Alcohol consumption in Punjab. Indian Journal of Psychiatry. 1978;**20**:212-216

[22] Jain V, Pradhan SK, Vibha. Socio-demographic profile of 15-24 years old male narcotic substance users in a resettlement colony of Delhi. Indian Journal of Public Health. 2009;**53**:44-47

[23] Barua A, Dasgupta S, Mitra B, Sherpa PC, Tirwa M. Alcoholism among adolescent students of Tadong in East Sikkim. Journal of Asian Scientific Research. 2013;**3**(11):1105-1108

[24] Rehm J, Marmet S, Anderson P, Gual A, Kraus L, Nutt DJ, et al. Defining substance use disorders: Do we really need more than heavy use? Alcohol and alcoholism(Oxford, Oxfordshire). 2013;**48**(6):633-640. DOI: 10.1093/alcalc/agt127

[25] Jasani PK et al. International Journal of Community Med Public Health. 2019;**6**(5):1970-1974

[26] Weinberg NZ, Rahdert E, Colliver JD, Glantz MD, et al. Adolescent substance abuse: A review of the past 10 years. Journal of the American Academy of Child and Adolescent Psychiatry. 1998;**37**:252-261

[27] Juyal R, Bansal R, Kishore S, Negi KS, Chandra R, Semwal J, et al. Substance use among intercollege students in district Dehradun. Indian Journal of Community Medicine. 2005;**31**(4):252-254

[28] Sinha DN, Gupta PC, Pednekar M. Tobacco use among students in Bihar (India). Indian Journal of Public Health. 2004;**48**(3):111-117

[29] Padhy GK, Das S, Sahu T, Parida S. Prevalence and cause of substance abuse among undergraduate medical college students. Indian Medical Gazette. 2014;**148**(8):276-282

[30] World Health Organization. Child Abuse and Neglect, WHO fact sheet, N151. Available at: www.who.int/inffs/en/fact_151.html. [Accessed: May 19, 2013]

[31] Hasin DS, O'Brien CP, Auriacombe M, Borges G, Bucholz K, Budney A, et al. DSM-5 criteria for substance use disorders: Recommendations and rationale. The American Journal of Psychiatry. 2013;**170**(8):834-851. DOI: 10.1176/appi.ajp.2013.12060782

Chapter 5

The Physiological Effect of Excessive Indulgence: Its Diagnosis, Treatment, and Prognosis

Anilendu Pramanik and Sayan Mondal

Abstract

Too much of anything is bad for health. In recent years we have been familiar with "Binge". It may be in the case of eating, drinking, or watching movies. Generation Z is very much affected by this way of living. This habit comes from indulgence. These indulgences come mainly from heredity factors, psychological conditions, dieting, peer pressure, etc. Studies show that some important features can be shared, including personality and emotional features such as neuroticism and urgency. Excessive indulgence can lead to physical and mental breakdowns. Interpersonal psychotherapy (IPT) is an effective specialty treatment for different disorders that leads to a healthy life. A continuous effort to identify the consequences of binge behaviours will also aid the development of the research field. We have to build a society free from excessive indulgence.

Keywords: binge, epidemiology, neuropsychological, risk factor, health promotion

1. Introduction

Self-pity and addiction are excessive indulgences. That is binge-eating, binge-drinking, and binge-watching. It's a tendency to a lot of food consumption in a short period. Drinking and watching are part of excessive indulgences when happening too fast for a long time, such as movies, web series, etc. Too much pleasure just like drugs. which makes people physically and mentally upset. As a result, bulimia, obesity, anxiety disorder, and stress at work are seen. These indulgences come from our genetics, family history other physiological conditions, dieting, body image issues, etc.

Binge drinking is consuming consecutive alcoholic beverages for a limited period on one or more occasions within the past six months [1]. We know that Alcohols are made from different ingredients and the main ingredient is grape juice. This grape juice is very useful for us when we drink it directly. Again, if we filter this grape juice and mix it with different chemical ingredients again and again then the liquid solution we create is known as alcohol. such as wine and whiskey. Wine and whiskey have no taste no matter what you call them. this is like s poison, when we drink it, it goes straight to the stomach. After entering the stomach, large amounts of Hydrochloric acid (HCL) are secreted from the inner membrane of the stomach which destroys the inner membrane and causes ulcers. These alcohol molecules repeatedly irritate the cell as they travel from the stomach to the duodenum, causing the cells to become tumours or cancerous. After digestion, these molecules are absorbed and passed through the liver which has to do extra work for metabolizing. This extra work destroys the cells in the liver and disrupts other functions of the liver. On the one hand, as its cells are formed, on the other hand, its metabolism is disrupted and leads to cholesterol levels increased in the liver, causing the liver to become fatty. It damages the liver cells and causes liver cirrhosis which results in death. After metabolism in the liver, some molecules are carried directly to the heart by the hepatic vein into the brain and stimulate the nerves in the brain. this nerve becomes irritated and creates a kind of resonance that compels a person to drink alcohol, resulting in the person becoming intoxicated. in this condition, the nerves become weak and depression occurs.

Binge eating is a tendency of eating more food than usual in a short period (within any two hours) and loss of control over eating during this time [1]. Many people are food lovers again, whether they are at home or the wedding house, from a restaurant to street food, they are busy consuming food and they eat more food in less time. As a result, they suffer from gas and heartburn which is increasing day by day. Foodborne illness affects at least 9% of the world's population. 9% of the US population, or 28.8 million Americans suffers from an eating disorder. Less than 6% of people with eating disorders are medically diagnosed as "underweight".

The digestive system starts working only when we smell or see food so we can feel the urge to eat during the intake of food, we eat through the mouth which passes through the esophagus to the stomach, and from the stomach to the small intestine to the large intestine then the stomach and liver secrete useful enzymes. When we eat large amounts of food together, the stomach becomes bloated, and the chances of gas are more likely because the secretion of HCL increases. As a result, the symptoms of heartburn begin. When there is more pressure than necessary on different parts of the body, various problems arise in the physiological process. Excessive intake of food increases the secretion of serotonin and melanin hormones, leading to fatigue and drowsiness, and disruption of daily activities. Nausea occurs because of overeating and disregard for the hormone leptin. This hormone sends a message to the brain about whether the stomach is full or not and also tells you how much to eat. Failure to follow these instructions can lead to overeating and other problems. So, it is important to take an adequate amount of food and keep yourself healthy.

"Binge-watching" is on the rise in India. More than one lakh people fall victim to it every year. Binge-watching India ranks first in the global index. It is a habit where people tend to watch entertaining or informative content for a long period called binge-watching [2]. It could be a television show. Entertainment consumes people as they feel energetic as they watch more episodes together. People who stay up late at night binge-watching have sleep problems of circadian rhythm that result in brain chemical imbalances and negative programming in the subconscious mind. So, binge-watching should be avoided at night.

One of the things that are floating in front of our eyes is the world-famous web series "money heist" which is observed on Netflix. In this web series, people are entertained a lot and wait for the next part or next session so people enjoy entertainment for a long time at once and become a continuous factor program. Now it has been seen that instead of binge-watching, it has become purge watching. This desire to see does not come from within the individual's mind but is manifested in him to see by those around him then it is called purge watching. If a person watches the binge day by day as a result people feel anxious and lonely. Some research has shown that watching this binge causes heart problems in humans.

So, we don't understand when our entertainment becomes an addiction, so we fall prey to bingeing. So, we don't understand when our entertainment becomes an addiction, so we fall prey to bingeing.

2. Background

The eating problems of adolescents range from mild to severe eating disorders. Incidence rates of anorexia nervosa have increased seen from 1955 to 1984 among 10–19 years old, but not among adults, and the reported prevalence rate for anorexia nervosa of 0.48% among girls 15–19 years old in the United States. This disorder is the third most common chronic condition among adolescent girls after obesity and asthma. Binge eating was first recognized in a 1959 article by psychiatrist Albert Stunkard. He described this disorder as eating behaviour with excessive eating at irregular times. He associated a meal episode with a late-night meal. Over time, the term "bulimia" came to be used regardless of whether binge eating was day or night. Before the 1950s, bulimia would not have been easy for the average person to engage in, even if they had a tendency or desire to do so. Eating large amounts of food at one time meant getting the money or means for multiple meals at once. As the standard of living in Western societies has improved and the availability of cheaply produced large quantities of food has increased, so has the incidence of bulimia nervosa. Cognitive Behavioural Therapy (CBT) In the 1960s, Dr. Aaron T. was started by Beck. Dr. Beck realizes that his patients have inner dialogue or thoughts that affect their emotions. CBT has since become a type of therapy used to treat a variety of conditions, including eating disorders. CBT is still considered one of the main treatments for binge eating disorders. Although binge eating is not officially classified at this time, many doctors have begun prescribing stimulants to help obese people. In the 1970s and early 80s, the culture focused more and more on thinness and the rise of the supermodel phenomenon. The ideal body image of women is getting thinner. As a result, anorexia nervosa continues to grow. Until 1986, the American Psychiatric Association (APA) did not mention BAD in the Diagnostic and Statistical Manual of Mental Disorders (DSM). Even then, this disorder was considered a sign of bulimia. Attitudes towards eating disorders began to change in the 1980s. Celebrities like Princess Diana started talking about their eating disorder. Many college campuses have begun to offer counselling services to students with various eating disorders. In the 1990s Dialectical behaviour therapy was introduced by Dr. Marsha Linehan. it was a greatly advanced therapy treatment for binge eating disorder. In 1993 a Cognitive Behavioural Therapy manual was conducted by Fairburn, Marcus, and Wilson. They have also been shown to be effective in treating obsessive-compulsive disorder (OCD) as well as other types of impulsive behaviour. A variety of serotonin inhibitors have been used since the 1990s to treat depression and anxiety. These are Paxil [3], Zoloft (1992 for depression and 1996 for OCD), Luvox [3], and Celexa (Cipramil was first released in Denmark in 1989 and then became available in the United States in 1998). In 1994, BED was included in DSM-4. The American Psychiatric Association specifically mentions bulimia. The National Association of Eating Disorders was founded in 2001. This is the largest non-profit organization that supports families and individuals with various eating disorders. During this time, there were various excellent eating disorder resources and organizations formed to provide education and support to people suffering from eating disorders. The Binge Eating Disorder Association (BEDA) was founded in 2008. The association is a national organization focused on the diagnosis, prevention, and treatment of bulimia nervosa. This was an important step in helping people get the help they needed. In 2008, the National Institutes of Health showed that milnacipran is effective in treating bulimia. This particular drug showed personal improvement after 8 weeks of use. In 2013, BED was officially approved by DSM-5. This is the first time that bulimia has been recognized as a separate disorder from other types of eating disorders. This was an important step in helping people get the help they needed. In 2015, the Food and Drug Administration (FDA) approved a new drug to treat bulimia. The drug Lisdexamfetamine dimesylate was marketed under the name Vyvanse. This particular drug was prescribed to treat moderate to severe bulimia. Previously used to treat ADHD. The drug is rapidly absorbed from the intestinal tract and converted to dextroamphetamine. One way an individual can help control bulimia is to maintain a constant supply of the neurotransmitter dopamine in the brain. Binge eating and binge eating may be associated with reward centers in the brain. In 2019, researchers and healthcare professionals are still learning how BED affects different people and which treatment options are best for each individual [3].

The 1940s and 1950s were periods of heavy drinking. In the 1945 film The Lost Weekend, in which Don Berman is described as a periodic alcoholic. But in the current discussion, heavy drinking at the event is considered bilateral drinking. In the 1990s, it was often associated with public disorder and the relationship between alcohol consumption among young people and fear. This change originated in 1970 with scientific and policy. Over the last 50 years, the general context of alcohol treatment has been written in the UK. The post-war history of alcohol policy in the United States has been explored through recent research, which has led to an overall change in the prevailing notion of alcohol use and abuse. This proves the use and abuse of alcohol in the 1950s. At first, it was far from an ethical model of alcoholism as the problem was a lack of will towards a disease model or a distinct lack of moral origin which considered the problem a medical condition requiring treatment. Second, away from the disease model, the approach to public health and epidemiology has seen a reunion of the problem, which stems from overall alcohol consumption. Aiming at the 1990s, with the reduction of damages and the change in the way community is protected, the concept of light convergence within a criminal justice framework has been envisioned [4].

The word "Binge" first appeared in the mid-eighteenth century, meaning "wet". The word "binge" was used for eating or drinking during the First World War. But while the term "binge-watching" was coined in 2013, it gained popularity in 2012 [5]. Netflix had thirteen episodes of the first season of "House of Cards" in 2013. These episodes were released simultaneously, resulting in multiple episodes instead of one episode per week for which 2013 was marked as the Vision Streaming Era. 2015's "binge-watching" was first announced by Collins's English Dictionary as the best word of the year. 73% of Americans admit to "seeing the dilemma" which lasts 3 hours and 5 minutes. 90% of millennials and 87% of gen-z people are hesitant. 40% of people are of those ages who, on average, watch six episodes of television together once they sit down. Another hand the coronavirus epidemic is responsible for increasing division. HBO, for example, increased by 65% on March 14, 2000. Sykes's survey in 2021 found that 38% of respondents directed three hours or more of the "hours" of content by video, and 48% of it was done on holidays. Nielsen's study found that adults spent 3–4 hours or more watching live or streaming TV, which led them to underestimate the use of TV [6].

3. Binge eating

In most cases, a person suffering from a binge-eating disorder will consume large amounts of food. They will then feel unable to stop eating.

Although most people tend to overeat on occasion, some individuals have a hard time controlling their excessive consumption. This condition can lead to a binge-eating disorder.

Although most people suffering from binge-eating disorder are obese or overweight, they may also be at a normal weight.

3.1 Symptom

Some of the symptoms of this disorder include

- Large food consumption that occurs in a short period, such as over a couple of hours, can trigger feelings of being out of control.

- Some of the triggers that can trigger these feelings include overeating when you're not hungry, eating rapidly during a binge, or eating until you're full.

- Most people feel disgusted, ashamed, depressed, and anxious about their eating habits. They may also frequently diet without gaining weight.

After a binge, you don't compensate for the extra calories that you eat by exercising excessively, vomiting, or laxatives. This condition is similar to bulimia and restricting one's diet can lead to more binge eating.

The frequent episode of binging in one week defines the acute disorder.

If you or someone you know has a binge-eating disorder, please seek medical help immediately. Binge-eating problems can last for a long time, or they can be short-lived.

Binge-eating disorder can make it hard for others to detect its symptoms. Individuals with this condition tend to hide their behaviour, which can make it hard for others to identify them. If you think that a loved one may have the disorder, talk to them about it openly.

Support and encouragement can be provided to a loved one struggling with a binge-eating disorder. You can help them find a mental health professional and arrange an appointment.

3.2 Causes

Although it is not known why people with this disorder develop this condition, it is widely believed that various factors such as genetics, psychological issues, and long-term dieting can increase their risk of developing it. Binge-eating disorder can start in the late teens or early 20s.

Factors that may increase your risk of developing a binge eating disorder include:

Genetics: Individuals suffering from BED may have developed a heightened sensitivity to a chemical in the brain that's involved in feelings of pleasure and reward. It's also believed that the disorder is inherited [7–9].

A study conducted by Michigan State University revealed that there are genetic factors that can increase a person's risk of developing eating disorders. It looked at 500 female twins and found that environmental factors such as exposure to chemicals and alcohol before puberty were linked to the development of these disorders, but after puberty, the genetic factors were more prevalent [10].

The results of the study revealed that there could be a link between the presence of certain genes and eating disorders such as bulimia and anorexia. Further studies have also revealed that these disorders could be caused by a variety of genes [10].

Gender. In the US, 3.6% of women experience some form of bed at some point in their lives, which is higher than 2% of men. This is due to the biological factors that affect the development and maintenance of this condition [7, 11].

Compared to African-Americans, females were more prone to experiencing binge eating disorder (BED) and perceived discrimination. The link between perceived discrimination and the development of this condition was also stronger for males. The role of stressful life events and interpersonal issues in the development of this disorder has been known to affect the response of individuals with this condition [12].

Changes in the brain. There's a link between having a heightened response to food and having less self-control in people with BED [7].

The effects of aviation on the functioning of the neurotransmitters in the brain and the region of the brain that controls the movement of objects are known to be associated with the reduction in 5-hydroxytryptamine levels in individuals with an anxious temperament [13, 14].

Binge eating disorders and bulimia Nervosa are both characterized by episodes of binge eating. Various personality elements are related to these disorders, and the most common is impulsivity [15].

The negative urgency dimension exhibited by individuals with bulimia Nervosa and binge eating disorders is the strongest indication of their condition. This is because it triggers the activation of certain brain circuits that regulate reward and inhibitory control [16].

Body size. About 50% of people with Bedford have obesity, and 25% to 50% of those who seek weight loss surgery meet the disorder's criteria [8, 11, 17, 18].

Studies have shown that prolonged electroencephalographic (EEG) readings are associated with symptoms of eating disorders in individuals with higher BMI. These findings support the idea that neurocognitive reasoning plays a role in the development of effective interventions for individuals with eating disorders [19, 20].

Understanding the various mechanisms by which weight loss and gain occur can be influenced by studies on individuals with different weight disorders and populations. For instance, according to Feigel, athletes with spinal cord injuries are at risk of developing malnutrition and poor nutrition due to their sedentary lifestyle [21].

Body image. People with BED are prone to having a negative body image. This condition is caused by various factors such as overeating, dieting, and body dissatisfaction [22–24].

Binge eating. Most people with BED have a history of binge eating, which is regarded as the disorder's first symptom. This behaviour occurred during the teenage years and childhood [7].

One of the most common eating disorders that are co-occurring is Binge eating disorder (BED), which is characterized by significant physical and mental comorbidity, life impairment, and psychopathology. There are various treatment options for this condition, such as cognitive-behavioural therapy and pharmacotherapy [25].

Emotional trauma. Events such as the death of a loved one, abuse, or separation from a family member are considered risk factors for people with BED [26–28].

The trauma experienced during the past can be a contributing factor to the development of eating disorders, especially those that are characterized by binge eating and bulimia nervosa. It can also lead to other psychological conditions such as borderline personality disorder [29].

Other psychological conditions. Almost 80% of people with BED have at least one psychological disorder. Some of these include depression, anxiety, bipolar disorder, and substance abuse [17].

Binge eating is a type of psychological condition that occurs when one consumes a large amount of food. It can be triggered by various factors such as stress, dieting, and negative feelings about one's body shape.

3.3 Diagnosis

Although some people may have occasional overeating at Thanksgiving or other events, it does not necessarily mean they have BED. It can start in the teens to early twenties, though it can also occur at any age. People with this condition need support to overcome it, and it can last for a long time [30].

To be diagnosed, a person must have binge-eating episodes for at least three months. The severity of the condition ranges from mild to extreme, with the latter having up to 14 episodes a week.

One of the most important characteristics of binge-eating disorder is not taking action to stop it. Unlike bulimia, people with this condition do not resort to laxatives or exercise to suppress their binges.

Binge-eating disorder is more common in women than men. It is also more common among men than other eating disorders [31].

You should also talk to a mental health professional or medical provider about your symptoms and feelings. If you're not ready to seek treatment, ask someone you trust to talk about what you're going through. Having a friend, a faith leader, or a teacher can help you get the help you need to successfully treat binge-eating disorder.

3.4 The health risks

Binge-eating disorder (BED) is associated with various health conditions. It can also lead to obesity and other related issues. The increase in calories that people consume during these episodes is known to be a contributing factor to this issue [17].

Obese people are more prone to developing various health conditions such as heart disease, stroke, diabetes, and cancer. However, it has also been known that those who have a binge-eating disorder are more prone to experiencing these conditions than those who do not have this condition [30, 32, 33].

Among the other conditions that can be associated with binge-eating disorder include sleep problems, irritable bowel syndrome, and asthma. In women, it can lead to issues such as pregnancy complications and fertility problems [30, 31, 34].

Studies have shown that individuals with a binge-eating disorder are more prone to experiencing difficulties in social interactions [35].

Individuals with a binge-eating disorder are also more prone to experiencing hospitalizations and emergency department visits. Compared to those without this condition, those with a binge-eating disorder are more likely to have outpatient care and hospitalizations [36].

3.5 The treatment options

The treatment plan for individuals with a binge-eating disorder can vary depending on the severity of the condition and the goals. It can also focus on various aspects of one's body image and mental health.

Various forms of therapy can be used for individuals with a binge-eating disorder, such as medication, cognitive behavioural therapy, and interpersonal psychotherapy. These can be done on a one-to-one basis or in a group setting.

Although some individuals require only one type of therapy, others may need to try various combinations to find the right treatment plan. A mental health professional can help individuals determine which type of therapy is right for them.

3.5.1 Cognitive behavioural therapy

One of the most common forms of therapy for individuals with a binge-eating disorder is cognitive behavioural therapy. This type of therapy focuses on the relationship between negative thoughts and feelings about food and body shape [37, 38].

After identifying the triggers that contribute to the development of negative emotions, strategies can then be developed to help individuals change their behaviour [37].

These strategies can help individuals set goals, develop healthy eating habits, and monitor their food intake. They can also encourage them to change their thoughts about weight and body image [38].

One of the most effective treatment methods for individuals with a binge-eating disorder is CBT. According to a study, after 20 sessions, almost 80% of the participants were no longer binge-eating. 59% of them were still able to complete one year [38].

Another type of treatment is self-help CBT, which is typically delivered through a manual. This type of therapy allows participants to work on their own, and it also provides additional support [38].

Self-help therapy is more accessible and cheaper than traditional therapy. It can also be done through apps and websites. It's also proven to be more effective than traditional CBT [39, 40].

3.5.2 Interpersonal psychotherapy

Interpersonal psychotherapy is a type of therapy that focuses on the idea that binge eating can help individuals cope with various issues, such as relationship conflicts and grief [38].

This type of therapy aims to identify the specific problem that contributes to the development of negative eating behaviour. It then makes constructive changes to help the affected individual improve their behaviour [37, 41].

This type of therapy can be done in a group setting or on a one-on-one basis with a trained therapist. It's also sometimes combined with CBT. There's strong evidence supporting the positive effects of this type of therapy on reducing the behaviour of binge-eaters [38].

3.5.3 Dialectical behaviour therapy

The goal of a DBT session is to help individuals develop a plan to manage their emotions and cope with negative experiences. This method teaches them how to regulate their responses so they can manage their anger and manage their daily life without overeating. The four key areas of this therapy are interpersonal effectiveness, emotion regulation, mindfulness, and distress tolerance [38].

A study conducted on 44 women with binge-eating disorders revealed that after completing therapy, almost 90% of them were able to stop their binge eating. However, after six months, only 56% of them were able to maintain their recovery [42].

There's still a lot of research to be done on the long-term effects of DBT and how it can be compared to other treatment methods such as IPT and CBT.

3.5.4 Weight loss therapy

DBT is a behavioural weight loss therapy that aims to help individuals lose weight and improve their body image. It involves gradually making healthy lifestyle changes and monitoring their food intake. It's also expected that participants lose around a pound per week [38].

Although weight loss therapy can help individuals improve their body image and reduce their risks of developing obesity, it's not as effective as other treatment methods such as IPT and CBT when it comes to stopping binge eating [38, 40, 43, 44].

Although it's not as effective as regular weight loss, behavioural weight loss therapy can still help individuals achieve short-term, moderate weight loss. This type of therapy can be beneficial for people who have not been able to successfully use other treatment methods [38, 40].

3.5.5 Medications

Although these drugs are commonly used to treat binge eating disorders, they are not as effective as traditional therapy.

Other drugs that can treat binge eating disorders include antiepileptics and antidepressants. Also, some of these are used for treating hyperactive disorders [37].

According to studies, drugs are more effective than placebos when it comes to treating binge eating disorders. These drugs are 48 percent effective compared to 28.5 percent for the placebo [45].

These drugs can also help individuals with binge eating disorders by reducing their symptoms of depression and their appetite. However, more studies are needed to confirm the long-term effects of these drugs [37, 45].

Side effects of these drugs can also include stomach problems, sleep disorders, headaches, and increased blood pressure [31].

Individuals with binge eating disorders might also be able to benefit from additional medications to treat other mental health conditions.

3.6 Overcome

Getting the help of a medical professional is the first step in treating a binge eating disorder. This individual can help determine the severity of the condition and recommend the appropriate treatment. Although CBT is the most common treatment for this disorder, other methods such as combination therapy or individual therapy can also be effective. In addition to making healthy lifestyle choices, it's important to maintain a balanced diet and exercise program.

- *Keep a food and mood diary.* Keeping a diary of these individuals to deduce a diet and mood that identifies personal triggers is portrayed as an important step in controlling a dilemma.

- *Practice mindfulness.* It helps to increase self-control and maintain self-acceptance. Which can help to increase awareness of the trigger [46–48].

- *Find someone to talk to*. It is extremely important to get support whether it is through a partner, family, a friend, a binge intake support group, or online. 2 Choose healthy foods. A high-protein healthy diet, a diet consisting of regular meals and whole foods will provide an essential nutrient to satisfy hunger [49].

- *Start the exercise.* Regular exercise is a brilliant method to reduce weight and improve body image which helps to control anxiety and mood [50, 51].

- *Enough sleep.* Sleep is an underlying therapy that is closely associated with the causes of high-calorie intake and irregular eating. People make it a habit to sleep 7–8 hours out of 24 hours [52, 53].

4. Binge drinking

Binge drinking is a preventable serious public health problem.

Binge drinking is one of the most common and costly problems in the United States. If a man drinks 5 or more drinks at a party, while a woman drinks 4 or more drinks at a party [54], then this work is considered binge drinking. The proportion of "alcoholic youth" drinking is higher than that of "alcoholic adults", increasing from 50% between the ages of 12 and 14 to 72% between the ages of 18 and 20 [55].

Some people only drink, and they will not have the disease of alcohol use.

Again, some people who consume alcohol, are associated with an increased risk of various diseases from alcohol.

But binge drinking is a harmful risk behavior related to serious injury or many diseases.

4.1 Binge drinking is common

In the United States, one in six adults consumes at least 25 percent of alcohol each week.

Binge drinking is an approach where excess alcohol is blamed and more than ninety percent of adults in the United States are responsible for excessive drinking. From 1993 to 2001, the number of binge drinking episodes among U.S. adults increased from about 1.2 billion to 1.5 billion [56].

Binge drinking is mainly seen in young people who are between 18 and 34 years old. In general, men drink twice as much as women.

Excessive drinking is more common in adults with higher family incomes.

There are some groups or states for whom binge drinking is not common, but they drink frequently, i.e., consume alcohol frequently and in large quantities.

4.2 The stages of alcohol use disorder

Alcohol use that turns into a use disorder develops in stages [57].

At-risk stage: When you are suffering from stress and depression and you think about how to get rid of it, then you choose alcohol as the only way to get rid of it and start drinking socially. As a result, you become addicted to alcohol by concentrating on alcohol consumption.

Early alcohol use disorder: In this session, you will secretly start thinking about alcohol because of your drinking mentality and you will move towards the blackout.

Mid-stage alcohol use disorder: At this stage, the level of your alcohol consumption goes out of your range. As a result, he got involved in various problems in his daily life. You can find out about the damage to your various organs through lab and scan tests.

End-stage alcohol use disorder: At this point, you give up all your happiness and comfort and focus only on drinking. Which is why you are slowly moving towards death with organ damage.

4.3 How many binge drinks are consumed?

One out of every four adults in the United States drinks alcohol and they drink at least eight drinks on the occasion of a binge.

In total,17.5 billion adults drink bean sprouts a year. Adults drink 467 binge drinks each year. Four out of every five drinks are drunk by men [58].

Most people 21 years of age or younger drink alcohol and they consume large amounts of alcohol. Forty-four percent of high school students drink eight or more drinks in a row [59, 60].

4.4 Binge drinking is associated with many health problems, including

Binge drinking is associated with many health problems such as Unintentional injuries were motor vehicle collisions, burns, alcohol, poisoning, homicide, suicide, intimate partner violence, sexually transmitted diseases, unintended pregnancy, poor pregnancy resulting in miscarriage, stillbirth Diseases, sudden infant death, chronic diseases such as hypertension, stroke, liver disease, breast cancer seen in women, liver, colon, rectum, mouth, pharynx, and esophagus, including memory and learning problems, etc.

4.5 Effects of binge drinking on the developing brain ailments

Binge drinking is a pattern of alcohol drinking those results in a .08% alcohol concentration in a person's blood. The amount of alcohol consumed is five alcoholic drinks for men and four alcoholic drinks for women in about 120 minutes. This binge drinking occurs mainly in adolescents and young adults because they are taking heavy drinking with high frequency (i.e., 5 or more days in the past 30 days).

Neuron maturation occurs during the development of puberty that young adults are passing through. Magnetic resonance imaging has reported linear and nonlinear changes in Gray-matter and white-matter volume and thickness during development [54].

Both Gray matter and cortical Gray matter volumes decrease during adolescence when they are affected by binge drinking [61, 62]. Because of the low amount of Gray matter in the brain, which is related to Alzheimer's disease, depression, and post-traumatic stress disorder [63]. Although some studies have shown an increase in Gray-matter volume or thickness in binge drinks in adolescents, by the concomitant marijuana effect [64, 65]. If Gray matter increases the density it helps to higher processing and also increases mental development [66].

Other hands the development increase of white matter volume many times perceive in adolescence who binge drink. The microstructure of white matter has mixed results showing increased and decreased fractional anisotropy. Binge drinkers could lead to low task performance because of the risk of phenotype and inhibition of memory response during decision-making and reward response.

So, bring drinking effected on functional and anatomical changes in the brain. These are given below.

Adolescents and young adults' replication of binge drinking.		
Different parts of the brain	**Decreased/smaller**	**Increased/greater**
Frontal lobe	Gray-matter volume. Cortical thickness. Fractional anisotropy. Task activation: risk-taking/ reward response. Task activation: inhibition.	Task activation: working memory. Task activation: inhibition.
Striatum	Fractional anisotropy. Task activation: inhibition.	Task activation: cue reactivity.
Temporal lobe	Gray-matter volume. Fractional anisotropy. Task activation: verbal encoding.	Task activation: working memory and cue reactivity.
Cerebellum	Gray-matter volume. White-matter volume. Fractional anisotropy.	Task activation: working memory.
Occipital lobe	Fractional anisotropy.	Gray-matter volume.
Parietal lobe	Fractional anisotropy. Task activation: verbal encoding and inhibition.	Task activation: working memory. Task activation: verbal encoding and inhibition
Cingulate	Cortical thickness.	Nil

In the United States in 2014, 1.5 million adolescents (ages 12 to 17) and 13.2 million young adults (ages 18 to 25) were addicted to alcohol, with a percentage of 6.1% and 37.7%. 257,000 adolescents and 3.8 million young adults reported that they drank large amounts of alcohol and their percentage of 1 % and 10.8%. in the National Survey on Drug Use and Health.

4.6 Prevention of binge drinking

Binge drinking can be deadly in itself and may lead to an Alcohol Use Disorder (AUD). Take steps to cut down or abstain from alcohol before it seriously impacts your life. Here are five ways how to stop binge drinking.

4.6.1 Make a plan and put it in writing

Make a specific plan and write it down in a little notebook. Write down the causes of alcohol consumption and focus on gradual withdrawal. Record and look at the possible consequences of the various dangerous problems caused by the chemical poisoning of alcohol in the brain. If you feel like drinking, be aware of how much you are drinking or your condition. As a result, you can better diagnose your triggers and avoid the risk of foolish drinking.

4.6.2 Change your environment

Control the triggers of your drinking habits by eliminating the people, places, and events that lead to binge drinking. Games like "Beer Pong" or "Quarters" force you to drink too fast, so you don't realize how much you're drinking. Limit yourself to certain rules and drink non-alcoholic beverages.

4.6.3 Rely on family and friends for support

Create the mentality of staying away from or reducing alcohol consumption. There are some "accountability buddies" in your standardized support system who drink very little or no alcohol to help stop binge drinking. This helps prevent your trigger or depression. Even before planning an event where alcohol will be present. But with you comes a faithful aid as well as alcohol.

4.6.4 Abstinence may be your best approach

This is a simple and appropriate method were trying to abstain from alcohol or reduce its use. Alcohol use disorder AUD. It has symptoms and educates yourself about it. Join local alcoholic anonymous meetings and other alcohol support groups for valuable information. Which can prevent excessive drinking.

4.6.5 Ask yourself why you drink excessively

A therapist is needed to help you reduce stress, anxiety, loneliness, or other negative feelings, or to help you choose healthy ways to deal with feelings of being socially more comfortable. Make life easier by applying positive lifestyle changes, such as regular physical activity, eating nutritious food, participating in exciting sports or hobbies, and engaging yourself in alcohol-free events. Studies have shown that limiting yoga, mindfulness, inspirational reading, positive self-talk, negative news or TV shows, and spending time with positive thinkers improve self-esteem, mood, and long-term restraint. If it seems that AUG has an effect, take the medicine with the advice of a doctor who can prevent the disease.

5. Binge watching

The rise of binge-watching is becoming more common due to the COVID-19 pandemic. It can affect the body's energy balance and cause stress [67]. Binge-watching is a type of entertainment that occurs when people spend a lot of time watching TV. Although it's usually related to the show, there are concerns about its negative effects [68].

According to a study conducted by Sung et al., about 3 out of 4 of the respondents admitted to being binge viewers. In addition, research revealed that about 70% of TV viewers between the age of 13 and 49 consume at least one episode of a show at a time [69]. The term binge viewing refers to an excessive amount of television viewing. It has been known that media consumption can lead to various health conditions, such as depression and anxiety. In addition, viewers who binged on TV were more prone to experiencing loneliness and depression [70].

Today, most households in the US use a streaming service, and the amount of time they spend watching TV has drastically changed. Also, the rise of the Internet has increased the amount of time that college students spend watching TV [71].

Binge-watching is a type of entertainment that occurs when people spend a lot of time watching TV. It can be described as consuming at least two episodes of a particular series in one sitting. The length and number of these episodes are both referred to [72].

5.1 Binge-watching is like a drug

It's widely known that binge-watching TV shows can produce a high. Dopamine is a chemical that helps us feel good, and it's produced by our brain when we're engaged in an enjoyable activity. The release of this chemical helps us feel good, and it's similar to the effects of drugs and other substances that are addictive. As long as you continue to watch TV shows, your brain will continue to produce this chemical [73].

According to a survey conducted by Netflix, 73% of the people who binge-watched said they felt positive about their experience. According to psychiatrist Danesh A. Ali, a psychiatrist at North-western Medicine, repeated exposure to certain behaviours and thoughts can create neural patterns that are hard to break [74].

The effects of marathon viewing can have detrimental effects on your relationships and goals. It can make you feel irritable, defensive, and unreasonable if you're asked to stop, and it can even lead to you lying to cover up your binge. You may also find yourself constantly increasing the amount of time that you spend watching TV.

5.2 Health concerns

5.2.1 Binge-watching leads to mental health issues

Binge-watchers are more prone to experiencing depression and anxiety. They also reportedly have less self-control. One of the researchers, Yoon Hi Sung, said that viewers might start to neglect their relationships with others as a result of the increasing number of binge-watching [68, 75].

The same pathways that lead to sex addiction and heroin addiction are the same ones that trigger addiction to binge-watching. The body can become addicted to substances or activities that produce dopamine, which is a chemical that's involved in pleasure [73].

Excessive TV watching is linked to feelings of guilt, regret, and failure. After a binge-watching session, the viewers are more likely to feel depressed and anxious once the show has already ended. People might think that they will feel better if they're watching TV or some type of entertainment. They will feel more stressed out if they're binge-watching.

5.2.2 Binge-watching makes the show less fulfilling

Binge-watching revealed that people who watched several episodes of a show in one sitting were less likely to enjoy it. According to Damon Lindelöf, the co-creator of the show Lost, the concept of anticipation does not exist in binge culture.

Due to the popularity of binge-watching, it has become difficult for people who have not finished a new season to avoid spoilers on social media. Also, the lack of agreement regarding when the embargo should be lifted can cause conflicts among fans.

5.2.3 Binge-watching can cause serious physical health problems

It has been known that prolonged sitting can lead to various health conditions such as heart disease, cancer, and blood clots. People who are prone to binge-watching are also more likely to eat unhealthy food and gain weight.

People who binge-watch TV shows are more prone to experiencing fatigue and poor sleep quality. They also reportedly have higher chances of dying early.

Heavy users reported poor health-related characteristics and the unhealthiest dietary habits. Binge-watching was also associated with a higher likelihood of consuming fast food and having family meals in front of a TV.

5.2.4 Binge-watching leads to back problems

One of the most important factors that contribute to a healthy life is the spine. Unfortunately, many people who watch TV while sitting on their knees are prone to developing poor posture and experiencing back pain [76]. When people watch TV for a long time, their posture becomes curved, which makes them feel more comfortable. However, if it lingers too long, the smooth and balanced limbs become compressed, which can cause pain.

5.2.5 Binge-watching leads to respiratory function issues

The position of the body can affect the function and strength of respiratory muscles in both healthy individuals and those with cardiopulmonary dysfunction. For instance, young adults have less respiratory pressure and dyspnoea in the semi recumbent or supine position. On the other hand, the strength of their respiratory muscles is decreased in the supine position [77–81].

The length of a muscle fibres relationship with its surrounding tissues is biomechanically related to its ability to develop tension. It is believed that rib changes can affect the length-tension relationship of certain respiratory muscles, such as those in the diaphragm. This could cause these muscles to develop less tension and reduce respiratory rate [77, 82].

5.2.6 Lack of physical activity

If you spend your life lying on a cot without physical activity, you will be more likely to move towards heart disease with stroke [83].

The more often you watch TV, the softer you become, and the less likely you are to exercise for less than an hour. Six years of research show that more than 40% of adults over 15,000 are less likely to exercise.

5.2.7 Effect on brain

Researchers at Brigham and Women's Hospital recently discovered that falling asleep in front of a fluorescent light (about four hours) before going to bed results in less sleep, less REM sleep, and grogginess the next day, even after eight hours. The TV emits blue light that inhibits the release of melatonin, a hormone that helps you knock off [84].

5.2.8 Effect on the cardiovascular system

A type of disease that affects the blood vessels, cardiovascular disease (CVD) is a group of conditions that include heart failure, stroke, high blood pressure, atherosclerosis, and coronary artery disease [85]. People with CVD also have other conditions such as obesity, high glucose, smoking, and lack of exercise.

Worldwide, around 17.9 million people died due to CVD in 2015. In China, it has been reported that cardiovascular disease is the leading cause of death among the over-60 population [86]. Some of the risk factors that can contribute to this condition include being overweight, having diabetes, high blood pressure, and metabolic syndrome.

5.3 Managing binge-watching

- Limit yourself to a certain short episode beforehand, such as two or three episodes at a time then postpone watching TV and focus on some other work.

- Limits TV viewing levels by setting a low-timed episode

- Engage with other activities and balance them out, such as physical exercises, meeting and chatting with friends and reading, spending time with family, and indulging in social activities.

- Set a plan to watch only one show, but if you sit and watch the whole season at once, then this disorder will take time to re-evaluate.

5.4 Binge-watching is closely associated with sleep

Aside from affecting melatonin production, screen exposure can also affect sleep by interfering with the arousal response [87]. In studies, it has been shown that playing video games can increase activity in the autonomic nervous system, which can lead to prolonged sleep onset [88–90]. Another study revealed that social media use can affect the latency of sleep [91].

Studies on binge-watching have suggested that arousal could be a mediator of sleep. These shows, which are usually very complex and intense, tend to have a strong narrative structure and develop complex characters. As a result, viewers who watched these types of shows were more likely to become immersed in the story. Because of the complexity of the stories and the high emotional involvement, it has been theorized that binge-watching can affect sleep by interfering with the arousal response.

6. Conclusion

Any habit has a great impact on our lives, whether that habit is good or bad for our health. These habits are first triggered psychologically in our brain and simultaneously found an effect in the body. Bad habits have not acceptable for our health, but we should pay more attention to good habits because of anything in excessive amounts. is not good for our health such as Binge eating, binge drinking, and binge watching are the things that make our brain happy but harm our body. Any habit that behaves like a drug, which sometimes causes scars. We do not cure it in any other way. So, there is a defined way to cure every habit and identify it to make our life healthy and normal.

> *"A habit cannot be tossed out the window; it must be coaxed down the stairs a step at a time."*
>
> *—Mark Twain*

Author details

Anilendu Pramanik* and Sayan Mondal
MYAS—GNDU Department of Sports Sciences and Medicine, Guru Nanak Dev University, Amritsar, Punjab, India

*Address all correspondence to: anilendu.myas@gndu.ac.in

References

[1] Ferriter C, Ray LA. Binge eating and binge drinking: An integrative review. Eating Behaviors. 2011;**12**(2):99-107

[2] Schweidel DA, Moe WW. Binge-watching and advertising. Journal of Marketing. 2016;**80**(5):1-19

[3] The History of Binge Eating Disorder | Oliver-Pyatt Center. 2022. Available from: https://www.oliverpyattcenters.com/binge-eating-disorder-history/

[4] Berridge V, Herring R, Thom B. Binge drinking: A confused concept and its contemporary history. Social History of Medicine. 2009;**22**(3):597-607

[5] Word of the Day Binge Watching. 2019. Available from: http://www.macmillandictionaryblog.com/binge-watching

[6] Pro and Con: Binge-Watching. 2022. Available from: https://www.britannica.com/

[7] Bakalar JL, Shank LM, Vannucci A, Radin RM, Tanofsky-Kraff M. Recent Advances in Developmental and Risk Factor Research on Eating Disorders. Current Psychiatry Reports. 2015;**17**(6):42

[8] Davis C. The epidemiology and genetics of binge eating disorder (BED). CNS Spectrums. 2015;**20**(6):522-529

[9] Bulik CM, Sullivan PF, Kendler KS. Genetic and environmental contributions to obesity and binge eating. International Journal of Eating Disorders. 2003;**33**(3):293-298

[10] Jacquelyn Ekern MS. Genetic Factors Behind Eating Disorders. EatingDisorderHope.Com, 2017. Available from: https://www.eatingdisorderhope.com/blog/genetic-factors-eating-disorders

[11] Smink FRE, Van Hoeken D, Hoek HW. Epidemiology of eating disorders: Incidence, prevalence and mortality rates. Current Psychiatry Reports. 2012;**14**(4):406-414

[12] Assari S. Perceived discrimination and binge eating disorder; gender difference in African Americans. Journal of Clinical Medicine. 2018;**7**(5):89

[13] Friederich HC, Walther S, Bendszus M, Biller A, Thomann P, Zeigermann S, et al. Grey matter abnormalities within cortico-limbic-striatal circuits in acute and weight-restored anorexia nervosa patients. NeuroImage. 2012;**59**(2):1106-1113

[14] Strober M. Pathologic fear conditioning and anorexia nervosa: On the search for novel paradigms. International Journal of Eating Disorders. 2004;**35**(4):504-508

[15] Steiger H, Richardson J, Schmitz N, Israel M, Bruce KR, Gauvin L. Trait-defined eating-disorder subtypes and history of childhood abuse. International Journal of Eating Disorders. 2010;**43**(5):428-432

[16] Bechara A. Decision making, impulse control and loss of willpower to resist drugs: A neurocognitive perspective. Nature Neuroscience. 2005;**8**(11):1458-1463

[17] Hudson JI, Hiripi E, Pope HG, Kessler RC. The prevalence and correlates of eating disorders in the national comorbidity survey replication. Biological Psychiatry. 2007;**61**(3):348-358

[18] Reas DL, Grilo CM. Timing and sequence of the onset of overweight, dieting, and binge eating in overweight patients with binge eating disorder. International Journal of Eating Disorders. 2007;**40**(2):165-170

[19] Edwards CG, Walk AM, Thompson SV, Mullen SP, Holscher HD, Khan NA. Disordered eating attitudes and behavioral and neuroelectric indices of cognitive flexibility in individuals with overweight and obesity. Nutrients. 2018;**10**(12):1902

[20] Schmidt R, Sebert C, Kösling C, Grunwald M, Hilbert A, Hübner C, et al. Neuropsychologicalandneurophysiological indicators of general and food-specific impulsivity in children with overweight and obesity: A pilot study. Nutrients. 2018;**10**(12):1983

[21] Figel K, Pritchett K, Pritchett R, Broad E. Energy and nutrient issues in athletes with spinal cord injury: Are they at risk for low energy availability? Nutrients. 2018;**10**(8):1078

[22] Legenbauer T, Vocks S, Betz S, Puigcerver MJB, Benecke A, Troje NF, et al. Differences in the nature of body image disturbances between female obese individuals with versus without a comorbid binge eating disorder: An exploratory study including static and dynamic aspects of body image. Behavior Modification. 2011;**35**(2):162-186

[23] Stice E, Gau JM, Rohde P, Shaw H. Risk factors that predict future onset of each DSM-5 eating disorder: Predictive specificity in high-risk adolescent females. Journal of Abnormal Psychology. 2017;**126**(1):38-51

[24] Pearl RL, White MA, Grilo CM. Overvaluation of shape and weight as a mediator between self-esteem and weight bias internalization among patients with binge eating disorder. Eating Behaviors. 2014;**15**(2):259-261

[25] Hilbert A. Binge-eating disorder. Psychiatric Clinics of North America. 2019;**42**(1):33-43

[26] Degortes D, Santonastaso P, Zanetti T, Tenconi E, Veronese A, Favaro A. Stressful life events and binge eating disorder. European Eating Disorders Review. 2014;**22**(5):378-382

[27] Allen KL, Byrne SM, Crosby RD. Distinguishing between risk factors for bulimia nervosa, binge eating disorder, and purging disorder. Journal of Youth and Adolescence. 2015;**44**(8):1580-1591

[28] Hilbert A, Pike KM, Goldschmidt AB, Wilfley DE, Fairburn CG, Dohm FA, et al. Risk factors across the eating disorders. Psychiatry Research. 2014;**220**(1-2):500-506

[29] Túry F, Kovács-Tóth B. The role of traumatization in eating disorders. Possible therapeutic modalities with special regard to cognitive behavioral methods. Psychiatria Hungarica : A Magyar Pszichiatriai Tarsasag Tudomanyos Folyoirata. 2019;**34**(4):419-425

[30] Kessler RC, Berglund PA, Chiu WT, Deitz AC, Hudson JI, Shahly V, et al. The prevalence and correlates of binge eating disorder in the World Health Organization World Mental Health Surveys. Biological Psychiatry. 2013;**73**(9):904-914

[31] Guerdjikova AI, Mori N, Casuto LS, McElroy SL. Binge eating disorder. Psychiatric Clinics of North America. 2017;**40**(2):255-266

[32] Mehler PS, Frank GKW, Mitchell JE. Medical comorbidity and medical complications associated with

binge-eating disorder. International Journal of Eating Disorders. 2016;**49**(3): 319-323

[33] Raevuori A, Suokas J, Haukka J, Gissler M, Linna M, Grainger M, et al. Highly increased risk of type 2 diabetes in patients with binge eating disorder and bulimia nervosa. International Journal of Eating Disorders. 2015;**48**(6):555-562

[34] Olguin P, Fuentes M, Gabler G, Guerdjikova AI, Keck PE, McElroy SL. Medical comorbidity of binge eating disorder. Eating and Weight Disorders. 2017;**22**(1):13-26

[35] Kornstein SG, Kunovac JL, Herman BK, Culpepper L. Recognizing binge-eating disorder in the clinical setting: A review of the literature. Primary Care Companion to the Journal of Clinical Psychiatry. 2016;**18**(3):1-9

[36] Ágh T, Kovács G, Supina D, Pawaskar M, Herman BK, Vokó Z, et al. A systematic review of the health-related quality of life and economic burdens of anorexia nervosa, bulimia nervosa, and binge eating disorder. Eating and Weight Disorders. 2016;**21**(3):353-364

[37] Brownley KA, Berkman ND, Peat CM, Lohr KN, Cullen KE, Bann CM, et al. Binge-eating disorder in adults a systematic review and meta-analysis. Annals of Internal Medicine. 2016;**165**(6):409-420

[38] Iacovino JM, Gredysa DM, Altman M, Wilfley DE. Psychological treatments for binge eating disorder. Current Psychiatry Reports. 2012;**14**(4):432-446

[39] Perkins SSJ, Murphy RR, Schmidt UU, Williams C. Self-help and guided self-help for eating disorders. Cochrane Database of Systematic Reviews. 2006:1-90

[40] Wilson GT. Treatment of binge eating disorder. Psychiatric Clinics of North America. 2011;**34**(4):773-783

[41] Markowitz JC, Weissman MM. Interpersonal psychotherapy: Principles and applications. World Psychiatry: Official Journal of the World Psychiatric Association (WPA). 2004;**3**(3):136-139

[42] Telch CF, Agras WS, Linehan MM. Dialectical behavior therapy for binge eating disorder. Journal of Consulting and Clinical Psychology. 2001;**69**(6):1061-1065

[43] Peat CM, Berkman ND, Lohr KN, Brownley KA, Bann CM, Cullen K, et al. Comparative effectiveness of treatments for binge-eating disorder: Systematic review and network meta-analysis. European Eating Disorders Review. 2017;**25**(5):317-328

[44] Vocks S, Tuschen-Caffier B, Pietrowsky R, Rustenbach SJ, Kersting A, Herpertz S. Meta-analysis of the effectiveness of psychological and pharmacological treatments for binge eating disorder. International Journal of Eating Disorders. 2010;**43**(3):205-217

[45] Reas DL, Grilo CM. Review and meta-analysis of pharmacotherapy for binge-eating disorder. Obesity. 2008;**16**(9):2024-2038

[46] Godfrey KM, Gallo LC, Afari N. Mindfulness-based interventions for binge eating: A systematic review and meta-analysis. Journal of Behavioral Medicine. 2015;**38**(2):348-362

[47] Baer RA, Fischer S, Huss DB. Mindfulness-based cognitive therapy applied to binge eating: A case study. Cognitive and Behavioral Practice. 2005;**12**(3):351-358

[48] Smith BW, Shelley BM, Leahigh L, Vanleit B. A preliminary study of the

effects of a modified mindfulness intervention on binge eating. Complementary Health Practice Review. 2006;**11**(3):133-143

[49] Cadzow RB, Servoss TJ. The association between perceived social support and health among patients at a free urban clinic. Journal of the National Medical Association. 2009;**101**(3):243-250

[50] Bakland M, Rosenvinge JH, Wynn R, Sundgot-Borgen J, Fostervold Mathisen T, Liabo K, et al. Patients' views on a new treatment for Bulimia nervosa and binge eating disorder combining physical exercise and dietary therapy (the PED-t). A qualitative study. Eating Disorders. 2019;**27**(6):503-520

[51] Larsen JK, Geenen R, Van Ramshorst B, Brand N, Hox JJ, Stroebe W, et al. Binge eating and exercise behavior after surgery for severe obesity: A structural equation model. International Journal of Eating Disorders. 2006;**39**(5):369-375

[52] Trace SE, Thornton LM, Runfola CD, Lichtenstein P, Pedersen NL, Bulik CM. Sleep problems are associated with binge eating in women. International Journal of Eating Disorders. 2012;**45**(5):695-703

[53] Dashti HS, Scheer FAJL, Jacques PF, Lamon-Fava S, Ordovás JM. Short sleep duration and dietary intake: Epidemiologic evidence, mechanisms, and health implications. Advances in Nutrition. 2015;**6**(6):648-659

[54] Jones SA, Lueras JM, Nagel BJ. Effects of binge drinking on the developing brain. Alcohol Research: Current Reviews. 2018;**39**(1):87-96

[55] Siqueira L, Smith VC. Binge drinking. Pediatrics. 2015;**136**(3):e718-e726

[56] Naimi TS, Brewer RD, Mokdad A, Denny C, Serdula MK, Marks JS. Binge drinking among US adults. Journal of the American Medical Association. 2003;**289**(1):70-75

[57] Svyatets K. Alcohol Use Disorder. 2022. pp. 21-31. DOI: 10.1007/978-3-030-86430-9_3

[58] Kanny D, Naimi TS, Liu Y, Lu H, Brewer RD. Annual total binge drinks consumed by U.S. Adults, 2015. American Journal of Preventive Medicine. 2018;**54**(4):486-496

[59] Jones CM, Clayton HB, Deputy NP, Roehler DR, Ko JY, Esser MB, et al. Prescription opioid misuse and use of alcohol and other substances among high school students – Youth risk behavior survey, United States, 2019. MMWR Supplements. 2020;**69**(1):38-46

[60] Esser MB, Clayton H, Demissie Z, Kanny D, Brewer RD. Current and binge drinking among high school students — United States, 1991-2015. MMWR. Morbidity and Mortality Weekly Report. 2017;**66**(18):474-478

[61] Pfefferbaum A, Rohlfing T, Pohl KM, Lane B, Chu W, Kwon D, et al. Adolescent development of cortical and white matter structure in the NCANDA sample: Role of sex, ethnicity, puberty, and alcohol drinking. Cerebral Cortex. 2016;**26**(10):4101-4121

[62] Mashhoon Y, Czerkawski C, Crowley DJ, Cohen-Gilbert JE, Sneider JT, Silveri MM. Binge alcohol consumption in emerging adults: Anterior cingulate cortical "thinness" is associated with alcohol use patterns. Alcoholism: Clinical and Experimental Research. 2014;**38**(7):1955-1964

[63] Cohut M. Action video games decrease gray matter, study finds.

Medical News Today. 2017. Available from: https://www.medicalnewstoday.com/articles/318839

[64] Jacobus J, Squeglia LM, Meruelo AD, Castro N, Brumback T, Giedd JN, et al. Cortical thickness in adolescent marijuana and alcohol users: A three-year prospective study from adolescence to young adulthood. Developmental Cognitive Neuroscience. 2015;**16**:101-109

[65] Jacobus J, Squeglia LM, Sorg SF, Nguyen-Louie TT, Tapert SF. Cortical thickness and neurocognition in adolescent marijuana and alcohol users following 28 days of monitored abstinence. Journal of Studies on Alcohol and Drugs. 2014;**75**(5):729-743

[66] Guy-Evans O. Grey matter vs white matter in the brain. Simply Psychology. 2021 Available from: https://www.spinalcord.com/blog/gray-matter-vs-white-matter-in-the-brain

[67] Aghababian AH, Sadler JR, Jansen E, Thapaliya G, Smith KR, Carnell S. Binge watching during covid-19: Associations with stress and body weight. Nutrients. 2021;**13**(10):3418

[68] Starosta J, Izydorczyk B, Wontorczyk A. Anxiety-depressive syndrome and binge-watching among young adults. Frontiers in Psychology. 2021;**12**:1-13

[69] Matrix S. The Netflix effect: Teens, binge watching, and on-demand digital media trends. Jeunesse: Young People, Texts, Cultures. 2014;**6**(1):119-138

[70] Exelmans L, Van Den Bulck J. Binge viewing, sleep, and the role of pre-sleep arousal. Journal of Clinical Sleep Medicine. 2017;**13**(8):1001-1008

[71] Damratoski KJ, Field AR, Mizell KN, Budden MC. An investigation into alternative television viewership habits of college students. Journal of Applied Business Research. 2011;**27**(1):69-76

[72] Flayelle M, Maurage P, Di Lorenzo KR, Vögele C, Gainsbury SM, Billieux J. Binge-watching: What do we know so far? A first systematic review of the evidence. Current Addiction Reports. 2020;**7**(1):44-60

[73] How Unhealthy Is Binge Watching? Press Pause, and Read On, Reader's Digest. 2017. Available from: https://www.rd.com/culture/binge-watching-unhealthy/

[74] Mccracken G. Netflix ' Declares ' Binge ' Watching ' is ' the ' New ' Normal (pp. 1-2). 2015. Available from: https://www.prnewswire.com/news-releases/netflix-declares-binge-watching-is-the-new-normal-235713431.html

[75] Sun JJ, Chang YJ. Associations of problematic binge-watching with depression, social interaction anxiety, and loneliness. International Journal of Environmental Research and Public Health. 2021;**18**(3):1-19

[76] How Binge-Watching TV Can Affect Spine Health. 2020. Available from: https://health.usnews.com/health-care/for-better/articles/how-binge-watching-tv-can-affect-spine-health

[77] Costa R, Almeida N, Ribeiro F. Body position influences the maximum inspiratory and expiratory mouth pressures of young healthy subjects. Physiotherapy (United Kingdom). 2015;**101**(2):239-241

[78] Badr C, Elkins MR, Ellis ER. The effect of body position on maximal expiratory pressure and flow. The Australian Journal of Physiotherapy. 2002;**48**(2):95-102

[79] Terson de Paleville DGL, Sayenko DG, Aslan SC, Folz RJ, McKay WB, Ovechkin AV. Respiratory motor function in seated and supine positions in individuals with chronic spinal cord injury. Respiratory Physiology & Neurobiology. 2014;**203**:9-14

[80] Melam GR, Buragadda S, Alhusaini A, Alghamdi MA, Alghamdi MS, Kaushal P. Effect of different positions on FVC and FEV1 measurements of asthmatic patients. Journal of Physical Therapy Science. 2014;**26**(4):591-593

[81] Koulouris N, Mulvey DA, Laroche CM, Goldstone J, Moxham J, Green M. The effect of posture and abdominal binding on respiratory pressures. European Respiratory Journal. 1989;**2**(10):961-965

[82] Cormie P, McGuigan MR, Newton RU. Developing maximal neuromuscular power: Part 1 - Biological basis of maximal power production. Sports Medicine. 2011;**41**(1):17-38

[83] Tian D, Meng J. Exercise for prevention and relief of cardiovascular disease: Prognoses, mechanisms, and approaches. Oxidative Medicine and Cellular Longevity. 2019;**2019**:3756750

[84] 6 Physical Effects of Binge-Watching TV. 2015. Available from: https://www.gq.com/story/tv-binge-watching-effects

[85] Yong J, Lin D, Tan X-R. Primary prevention of cardiovascular disease in older adults in China. World Journal of Clinical Cases. 2017;**5**(9):349

[86] Jiang Y, Mao F, Li Y, Liu J, Zhang Y, Jiang Y, et al. Construction of China cardiovascular health index. BMC Public Health. 2018;**18**(1):937

[87] Cain N, Gradisar M. Electronic media use and sleep in school-aged children and adolescents: A review. Sleep Medicine. 2010;**11**(8):735-742

[88] Dworak M, Schierl T, Bruns T, Strüder HK. Impact of singular excessive computer game and television exposure on sleep patterns and memory performance of school-aged children. Pediatrics. 2007;**120**(5):978-985

[89] Higuchi S, Motohashi Y, Liu Y, Maeda A. Effects of playing a computer game using a bright display on presleep physiological variables, sleep latency, slow wave sleep, and REM sleep. Journal of Sleep Research. 2005;**14**(3):267-273

[90] Ivarsson M, Anderson M, Åkerstedt T, Lindblad F. Playing a violent television game affects heart rate variability. Acta Paediatrica, International Journal of Paediatrics. 2009;**98**(1):166-172

[91] Harbard E, Allen NB, Trinder J, Bei B. What's keeping teenagers up? Prebedtime behaviors and actigraphy-assessed sleep over school and vacation. Journal of Adolescent Health. 2016;**58**(4):426-432

Chapter 6

The First Offer of Alcohol from the Adult Person and Cannabis Use

Alojz Nociar and Stanislava Šaffová

Abstract

This chapter is based on the data from the national survey on tobacco, alcohol, and drugs among primary and secondary school students aged 15–19 implemented in eight regions of Slovakia during Spring 2018. An unexpected shift was observed in the relationship between the age young people were offered alcohol by an adult and the age when they first experienced its effect. In previous surveys, the mean age of the first offer predated the felt effect of alcohol ("tipsiness") by about 1 year on average. Our data revealed that following the initial offer of alcohol by an adult, approximately ¾ of participants felt the effect of alcohol ***later*** or during the same year (groups 1 and 2); however, in the remaining cases, the effect was felt ***before*** alcohol was offered by an adult (group 3). Thus, it appears that one-fifth to one-quarter of participants did not go through the usual ritual of initiation by adults. The analysis showed that this group of participants used cannabis more often than the rest of the sample. Furthermore, there were differences observed among the three groups in reported school attendance, legal and illegal drug use, and bullying. Possible implications of these findings are discussed.

Keywords: age of the first offer, tipsiness before or after offer of alcohol, cannabis use, adult persons and drinking initiation

1. Introduction

In research focused on the first exposure to alcohol, the age of the initial contact with this substance is frequently used as a crucial variable potentially associated with future health and psychosocial problems connected to alcohol and drug dependency [1, 2]. However, less is known about the typical situations, contexts, and circumstances in which such first contact and early use of alcohol occur. Alcohol is often offered to young people by an adult in cultures with a permissive approach to this substance (in which it is often legalized and socially accepted). It is interesting that the use of legal drugs in early adolescence is considered as something obvious and even normal even in the countries where legislation does not permit underage drinking and tobacco smoking, and bans are in place for selling these products to minors and adolescents. Since minors do report the use of legal drugs in anonymous surveys, it is likely that alcohol beverages and tobacco products are offered to them by adults, most probably by close family members, relatives, older friends, or siblings. It would therefore seem a common sense to assume that asking about the age of the first offer of alcohol from an adult would be practically the same as asking for the age of the first drink.

Previous research aimed at differentiating between the age of the first contact with any sort of alcohol and the first experience of alcohol-induced changes in mood or psychological state demonstrated that the age of the first drink may be less important as an indicator of the future problems than the age of the first alcohol intoxication [3].

Some studies attempted to explain the use of legal and illegal drugs in early adolescence *via* specific micro-social conditions, adherence to traditions and different drinking cultures in various European countries is based on the geographical location [4], and other authors investigated whether this phenomenon might be caused by significant sociopolitical changes such as those happening in Europe after the fall of the so-called iron curtain, which divided the West from the Eastern European countries after 1989 [5].

Another research trend focused on the investigation of possible connections between legal and illegal drug use and antisocial behaviors at school (e.g., aggression or bullying). The researchers examined and highlighted the associations between bullying and the use of both legal and illegal drugs in those who perpetrated bullying as well as in the victims and bystanders. Other relevant psychological and social variables were included in their investigation [6–8]. Ake to boli napriklad tie variables?

Alcohol tends to be used as a socially tolerated drug throughout human life during special occasions and may be a common part of various cultural traditions. During such special occasions (e.g., name days, birthdays, Christmas, or New Year), the family tends to be the primary environment where children and adolescents may be offered alcohol by an important adult, which may model their future alcohol-related behaviors and attitudes (i.e., the social approval of underage drinking). For example, the studies using natural experiments demonstrated that pre-school children who were asked to pretend to act as adults during a birthday celebration started to pretend to be "drunk," likely imitating what they had previously seen [9].

We tried to find out more about these types of situations through two of the core questions of the TAD (Tobacco, Alcohol, Drugs) questionnaires. The data showed that the percentages of the children and adolescents to whom alcohol beverages were offered by adults during socially approved events seemed to be high and growing year after year as outlined in **Figures 1** and 2.

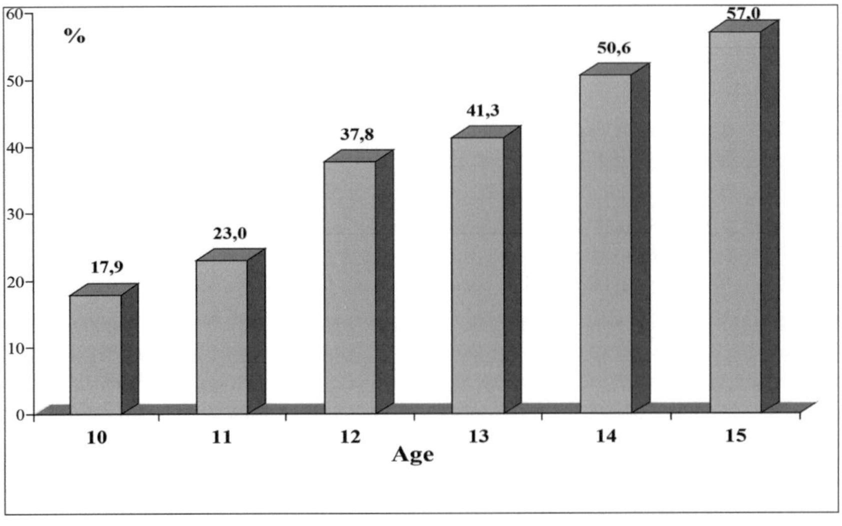

Figure 1.
Champagne wine offered by parents to their children as a new Year's toast (percentages in 2018).

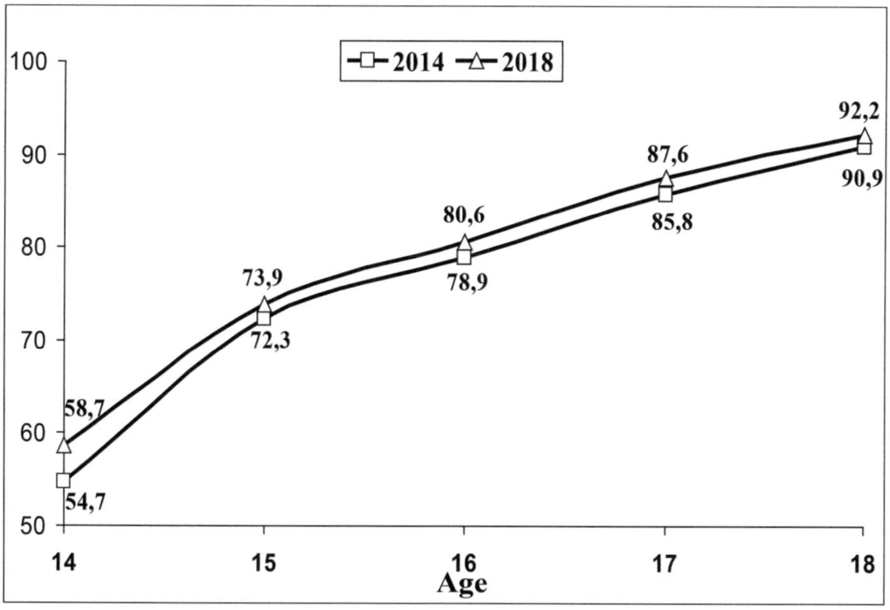

Figure 2.
Any alcohol offered to teens by adults for the first time (in percentages).

The data clearly demonstrated the annual increases in number of young people to whom alcohol beverages were offered by an adult during a socially approved event, while the average age of the first experience with the three main types of alcohol beverages was relatively constant (around an average of 10 years and growing very slowly)—please refer to **Figure 3**.

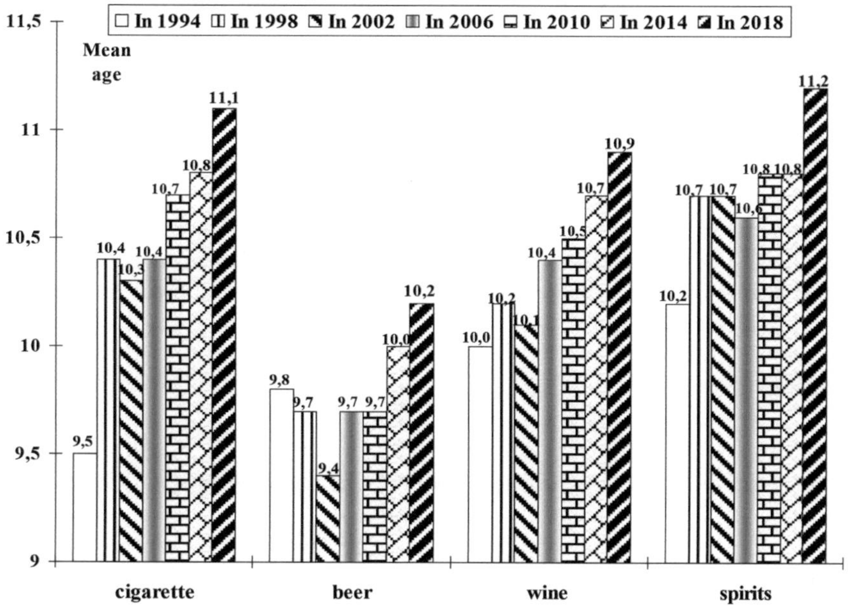

Figure 3.
Tobacco and alcohol used for the first time: 11–14 year olds.

2. Methods

Three TAD questionnaires were used to monitor the level of tobacco, alcohol, and drug use *via* surveys conducted in regular 4-yearly cycles from 1994 till 2018. The questionnaires were devised to map the impact of the nationwide drug prevention program "School without alcohol, nicotine and drugs" [10]. The questionnaires consisted of [number of questions]. The data from these surveys were processed by statistical package for social sciences (SPSS 20.0).

The surveys were carried out among primary school pupils from grades 5 to 9, aged 10–15 (TAD1). TAD1 questionnaires assessed 30 day, 12 months, and lifetime prevalence of drug use, together with the items on early start of drug use and family environment. The items on aggression and bullying at school were used from 2010 until 2018 [11].

A similar survey (TAD2) was carried out in secondary schools among 16–19 year olds. Apart from the traditional scheme of epidemiological information on drugs, bullying, and aggression, TAD2 contained items assessing the presence of alcohol dependence symptoms, namely screening CAGE (Cut down, Annoyed, Guilty, Eye-opener) and shortened ADS (Alcohol Dependence Scale—see [12, 13]).

Finally, TAD3 questionnaire was used asking for primary and secondary school teachers' own use of legal drugs such as tobacco and alcohol, knowledge about illegal drugs, as well as their attitudes toward and willingness to take part in school prevention programs.

All the above surveys were approved by the Ministry of Education of the Slovak republic, and the data collection was implemented by the Ministry of Health' network of the Slovak Office of Public Health in the whole country under the coordination of the first author.

From 1998, TAD2 questionnaire contained two items to capture at least some information related to the early start of the individual experience with alcohol; the questions remained unchanged in all TAD2 versions until 2018. They were as follows:

Did it happen, that adult person offered you to drink alcohol beverage?

1☐ No.

2☐ Yes → ***If yes,** 1st time it had happened, when I was **about:........years old.***

Have you ever felt, that you were somewhat "tipsy" (or "half drunk")?

1☐ No.

2☐ Yes → ***If yes,** 1st time it had happened, when I was **about:........years old.***

The last one from the seven anonymous surveys, from which the data for the purpose of this chapter were derived, was conducted in 2018 among 15–19 year olds (n = 4042; 2194 boys and 1848 girls) from ninth grades of the primary schools and from four grades of the secondary schools of all types from grammar and vocational schools in the Slovak republic [14].

2.1 Design and data

All TAD questionnaires were administered anonymously, and respondents received their paper-pencil versions, provided their answers without any personal data, which might be used to identity an individual, class, or school. Only the information about the year of birth and gender was required as obligatory to enable comparisons between boys and girls of certain age. Every respondent had right to refuse to take part in survey.

After completing, respondents returned filled questionnaires in sealed envelopes without any mark, except for the mark written by research assistants to the big envelope with encrypted code of class and school, assigned by survey coordinator. In the seven research waves, 32,814 primary school pupils, 29,375 secondary school students, and finally, 10,180 teachers from both types of schools participated in the surveys.

All three TAD questionnaires were used across the eight main regions of Slovakia, with their samples being self-weighted for gender, school, class, region, and teaching language, taking into account also minorities as the part of the selection criteria.

The samples were created by a stratified proportional random sampling from ninth grades of primary and first to fourth grades of secondary schools, from five types of schools (primary, secondary grammar schools lasting 4 and 8 years, then secondary specialized schools with and without maturity exams, i.e., those lasting from 4 to 5 years, and the secondary specialized schools lasting 3 years only), selected proportionally from eight main regions of the whole country.

The sampling unit was school, and within each selected secondary school, four classes were randomly selected by research assistants from the first to the fourth grades; and one class from each of the existing ninth grades in selected primary schools, because part of the cohort of 15–16 year olds was still in primary schools, while approximately ¾ of them were in the secondary schools, predominantly in the first grade.

The scope of selection was defined according to the requirement for reliability (95%) and preciseness (2%), with respect to the existing numbers of primary school pupils and secondary school students still attending schools in Slovakia and with respect to the age range to be covered, that is, from 15 to 16 to 18–19 year olds.

2.2 Results

At the beginning, we counted overall means of ages for offer and for effect in the same way as before, that is, for the whole sample. But during TAD2 data entries in 2018, we noticed frequent inconsistencies with previous results such as a younger age of the first experience of tipsiness than the age of alcohol offer. **Table 1** outlines the average ages for the first offer and the effect felt after any drinking of alcohol for TAD surveys from 1998 until 2018.

In previous surveys, the mean age at the two points mapped by TAD2 was calculated, as it is indicated in the table above. Averages for the whole dataset showed that the first offer of alcohol came earlier, while "tipsiness" felt subjectively for the first time was observed about 1 year later. However, closer inspection of the data in part of the cases had shown that the "tipsiness" occurred ***later*** or during the same year, but in

Year of TAD survey Mean age	**1998** n = 548	**2002** n = 3678	**2006** n = 4915	**2010** n = 3112	**2014** n = 2252	**2018** n = 1751
Alcohol offered by adult person for the first time	13,37	12,88	13,48	13,68	13,89	14,15
Effect of alcohol felt for the first time ("tipsiness")	14,21	14,51	14,62	14,52	14,55	15,08

Table 1.
Mean ages of the first offer of alcohol by an adult person and the age when the effect of alcohol was felt ("tipsiness").

some smaller, but still in substantial proportion of the cases, this effect of alcohol was reported as felt ***before*** any alcohol beverage was offered by an adult person.

In other words, approximately one-fifth to one-quarter of the adolescents did not go through the usual ritual of alcohol drinking initiation by adults; they appeared to try alcohol in their own way, not adhering to any symbolic adult permissions.

Thus, three groups were identified within this whole sample in respect to the age of alcohol beverage offer and the age of the pharmacological effect of alcohol upon mood and/or psychological state, felt for the first time in life:

1. offer and effect occurred ***during*** the same year;

2. effect occurred one or more years ***after*** the offer;

3. effect was experienced ***before*** the offer from an adult person.

The first two groups appeared to have acted in line with unwritten social rules of handling situations where alcohol is offered, that is, group 1 (no difference in the age, i.e., offer and effect in the same year), group 2 (effect delayed), and finally, the third group, where offer of alcohol from an adult was not related to the effect felt (which thus is unlikely to be associated with an adult offer) (**Figure 4**) [14].

These groups were then compared with respect to some of the variables from TAD2 surveys' results to find the possible differences in lifetime prevalence of cannabis. There were no significant differences in numbers of boys and girls in any of these three groups.

As we might see, the third group differed from first and second groups in higher proportion of cannabis lifetime use (**Table 2**), in this case characterized by an almost reverse percentages of cannabis lifetime prevalence. And roughly similar third groups were identified also in the series of previous TAD2 surveys, as well as across the teenage period (**Table 3**).

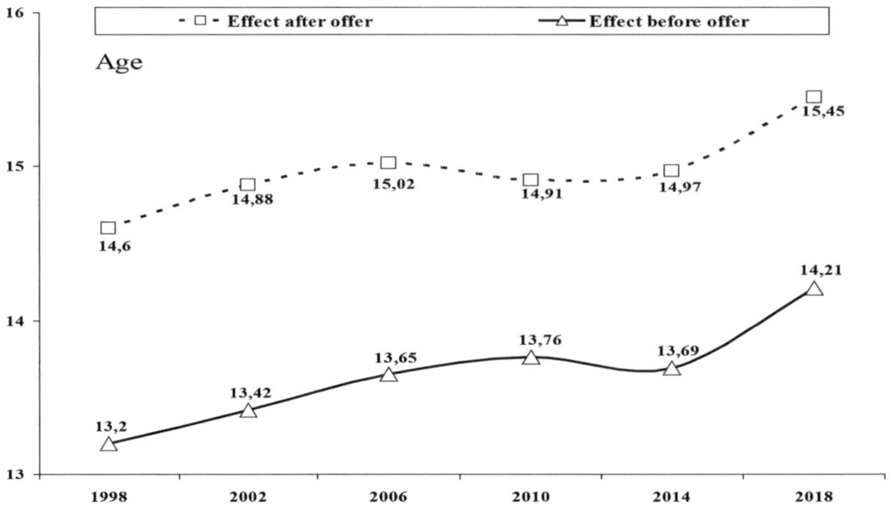

Figure 4.
Average ages of the first experience with alcohol effect ("tipsiness"): **After** *offer of alcohol; and* **before** *offer of alcohol by adult person.*

		Effect_Before_After variable			Total
		1st group	**2nd group**	**3rd group**	
		Offer & effect in the same age	**Tipsiness after Adult Offer**	**Tipsiness before Adult Offer**	
Did you ever smoked marihuana or used hashish?	**YES**	n = 260	n = 370	n = 204	n = 834
		41,3%	37,8%	**61,6%**	43,0%
	NO	n = 370	n = 608	n = 127	n = 1105
		58,7%	62,2%	**38,4%**	57,0%
Total		n = 630	n = 978	n = 331	n = 1939
		100,0%	100,0%	100,0%	100,0%

Table 2.
Cannabis use differences between three groups of respondents in TAD2 2018 survey (Chi² significant at 0,000).

	Effect_Before_After variable											
	1st group				**2nd group**				**3rd group**			
	Offer & effect in the same age				**Tipsiness after Adult Offer**				**Tipsiness before Adult Offer**			
Students from 16 to 19 years:	16	17	18	19	16	17	18	19	16	17	18	19
YES	37,0	47,4	46,9	43,8	33,9	37,1	37,9	37,1	47,2	71,6	58,6	67,3
Did you ever smoked cannabis or used hashish? **NO**	63,0	52,6	51,3	56,2	66,1	62,9	62,1	62,9	52,8	28,4	41,4	32,7

Table 3.
Cannabis lifetime prevalence in three groups differing in the age of alcohol offer and tipsiness effects sorted by age from 16 to 19.

The relationship between cannabis use and the tipsiness experienced before an adult offer of alcohol did not appear to be incidental as it was observable not only in the year of the last implemented TAD2 survey, but also across all surveys from 1998 till 2018. This was an interesting finding, and we wondered whether these differences of the third group from two others might be related to other variables, such as parental control, family status, school attendance, or others.

Therefore, we decided to use the two questions about the offer and the tipsiness in a forthcoming broader survey implemented across Europe, namely the ESPAD project during the Spring 2019 [9]. (See **Table 4**).

The results outlined in **Table 4** appear to confirm the trend revealed by TAD2 survey implemented in 2018: the third group as documented in ESPAD survey carried out 1 year later (n = 9338) was different from the two other groups in lifetime prevalence of cannabis use, even though these results were not fully identical.

As there are likely to be additional variables relevant to this problem, we tried to map some of them within our existing datasets. Even though our surveys, both TAD and ESPAD, were not specifically designed to examine this problem (early experience with alcohol and its subjectively felt pharmacological effect), we decided to map at least some of the variables such as the important persons from the family

		Effect_Before_After variable			Total
		1st group	**2nd group**	**3rd group**	
		Offer & effect in the same age	**Tipsiness after Adult Offer**	**Tipsiness before Adult Offer**	
Did you ever smoked marihuana or used hashish?	**YES**	n = 536	n = 754	n = 594	n = 1884
		41,6%	38,2%	**63,9%**	44,9%
	NO	n = 752	n = 1221	n = 336	n = 2309
		58,4%	61,8%	**36,1%**	55,1%
Total		n = 1228	n = 1975	n = 930	n = 4193
		100,0%	100,0%	100,0%	100,0%

Table 4.
Cannabis use in three groups of respondents in ESPAD 2019 survey differing in the age of alcohol offer and tipsiness (Chi2 significant at 0,000).

environment, peers, older friends, classmates, or other people, as well as relevant events from close social environments of adolescents.

We tried to map the following variables:

1. School attendance

2. Legal and illegal drugs use

3. Alcohol abuse and related problems

4. Cannabis use related problems

5. Bullying and aggression at school

The third group, which appeared to have a tendency to circumvent accepted social norms and conventions about the initiation and/or the entrance into the adult community, was different from the two other groups also in other variables, not only in cannabis use prevalence (and it seems at the same time, that those variables were relatively less socially desirable).

In our preliminary analysis, we examined the variables such as school attendance with three main reasons of missing at school (see **Table 5**).

As for drugs use, the second and the third group were compared by nonparametric tests, and only results indicating significant differences are included in **Table 6**:

As for alcohol and related problems, except of usual core questions on prevalence (lifetime, 12 months, and 30 days), we also used a separate module with 30 items, containing two screening scales—CAGE and ADS [12–14].

Finally, cannabis-related problems were mapped by the items of CAST, used regularly in the ESPAD survey [15, 16]—see **Figure 5**:

Cutoff point, that is, point indicating case finding for CAST (which is 7 points) [17], we have found significantly higher number of the third group members, reporting more cannabis-use-related problems compared to group 1 and 2% (Chi^2 significant at 0.000).

		Effect_Before_After variable			Chi^2
		1st group	**2nd group**	**3rd group**	
		Offer & effect in the same age	**Tipsiness after Adult Offer**	**Tipsiness before Adult Offer**	
Missing at school because of:	***Illness***	58,9%	60,4%	56,9%	,056
	Truancy	***34,2%***	***33,1%***	***42,1%***	***0,001***
	Something else	60,8%	62,2%	62,8%	,229

Table 5.
School attendance in three groups differing in the age of the first offer of alcohol and in the age of the first tipsiness felt in the ESPAD2019 survey.

Question in TAD2(*), or questions in ESPAD (**)	**Effect_after_offer**	**Effect_before_offer**	**Chi^2**
Smoking cigarette at least once during lifetime*	65,2	86,9	0,000
Occasional smoking (1–2 cigarettes per month)*	36,8	61,7	0,000
Regular smoking (1–3 and more cigarettes per day)*	22,9	41,2	0,000
Hard drunkenness with the occurrence of palimpsests*	49,1	68,1	0,000
Lifetime use of ecstasy*	6,8	12,1	0,001
Lifetime use of LSD or hallucinogens*	3,4	7,9	0,000
C A G E**	0,83	0,92	0,40
A D S**	7,70	8,65	0,010

Table 6.
Legal and illegal drugs and related problems.

Only one from the items mapping aggression and bullying at school had shown significant difference in comparison of three groups:

He/she took part when group of his/her friends attacked other group.

Offer before Effect: (Chi^2 significant at 0.05);

As for items mapping group differences in perceived risk of drug use:

Five or more drinks every weekend—great perceived risk.

Offer before Effect: 54.3%; Effect before Offer: 47.3% (Chi^2 significant at 0,000).

Regular smoking of marihuana—great perceived risk.

Offer before Effect: 49.0%; Effect before Offer: 40.2% (Chi^2 significant at 0,000).

As for items mapping risky or hazardous behavior, like gambling:

He/she played for money—once monthly to 2–3 times weekly.

Offer before Effect: 15.3%; Effect before Offer: 21.0% (Chi^2 significant at 0,000).

He/she played for money on slot-machines—once monthly to 2–3 times weekly.

Offer before Effect: 5.1%; Effect before Offer: 9.9% (Chi^2 significant at 0,000).

Finally, the last items estimated a level of parental control:

His/her parents are setting rules on what I can do outside—almost never.

Offer before Effect: 36.4%; Effect before Offer: 44.2% (Chi^2 significant at 0,000).

His/her parents do know where he/she is at Saturday evenings—usually they do not.

Offer before Effect: 4.6%; Effect before Offer: 5.4% (Chi^2 significant at 0.023).

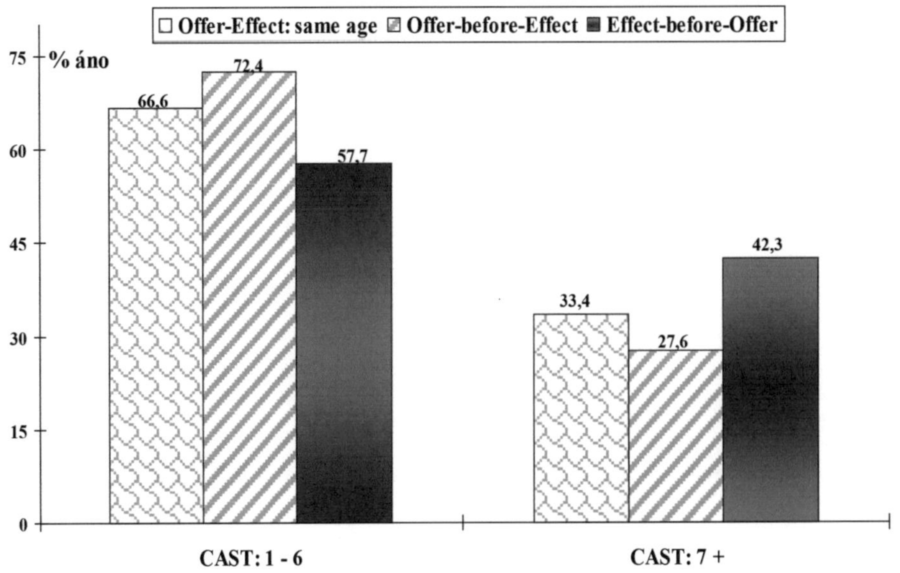

Figure 5.
The results of the CAST screening – Problems with cannabis use.

3. Conclusions

In previous surveys, the mean age at two points was calculated for the whole sample, and the first offer of alcohol came earlier on average, while the effect of alcohol (i.e. being "tipsy" or "half drunk") felt subjectively for the first time was observed around 1 year later. However, closer inspection of the data from 2018 survey revealed that in circa ¾ of the cases the effect occurred either ***later*** (mean age = 15.45) or during the same year (mean age = 14.94), but in the rest of the cases, this effect was felt ***before*** alcohol was offered by an adult person (mean age = 14.21).

Thus, around one-fifth to one-quarter of teens circumvented common ritual of alcohol drinking initiation by adults, and they have tried to do it their own way, not adhering to any symbolic adult permissions. Subsequent analysis had shown that this group not only has used cannabis more often than the rest of our sample, but there were also differences in other variables, such as school attendance, parental control, group aggression, and legal and illegal drug use.

These findings are consistent with several studies, where regular or even daily use of tobacco and alcohol was connected to the presence of risk behaviors correlated with early start of cannabis use by 15-year-olds or less, and this was even more intensive when such an early initiation had happened even earlier—in the age of 13 or less [18].

Perhaps some conclusions and recommendations might be eventually formulated. But at the moment, it would be not possible to define clear and rigorous facts with relevant explanatory power—our study was only mapping one part of a broad problem—how teens do start to form their drinking, smoking, and later on sometimes also drug taking habits. Together with other sorts of behaviors, which are, so to say, not very socially desirable—such as truancy, aggression, breaking accepted rules. All that taking place in social environment is now more than ever changing very rapidly with many unexpected and global changes and challenges.

If there would be some interest to investigate this problem in the future more deeply, planning of data gathering and introducing of relevant variables should take into account quite concrete matters—like how to ask appropriate questions about important others from family narrow environment, but maybe also broader environment such as districts or communities, social occasions where such an offer of alcohol from adult persons might came, and then types of such persons, such as peers of perhaps older siblings, etc.

Small preliminary attempts were already made also at our school *via* several bachelor theses [19], with some results indicating that the offer of alcohol by adult person occurred typically during family events, where mostly father, less frequently grandfather, or uncle has played active role in these processes, while females were involved also, but very rarely, in comparison with males. On the other hand, there were also indications of more frequent offers during less formal social events than social events within the family used to be—with offer of alcohol from older friends, peers, or sometimes from siblings.

So the main findings of this study on the distribution of the sample according to the age on an offer and effect of alcohol might be summarized as follows:

1. First two groups differed clearly from the third group in the lower occurrence of cannabis use.

2. This third group has had also higher use of tobacco.

3. The same is true for alcohol—also in simultaneously used CAGE screening and ADS scale.

4. This third group was also higher in illegal drug use—also in CAST screening targeted at problems connected with cannabis use.

5. This third group was different also in socially less desirable behaviors, such as truancy or group aggression.

6. This third group was trying to stay more or less out of parental control.

7. Perceived risk of drug taking was much lower in this third group, which has displayed a tendency to engage in gaming and gambling.

8. And finally, in spite of delineation of some personality traits in this group, we cannot say anything conclusive—also because of the fact that in this case, quantitative study with its rules and requirements, like those of anonymity, is reaching its limits and needs to be complemented perhaps by complementary qualitative studies.

Conflict of interest

The authors declare no conflict of interest.

Author details

Alojz Nociar* and Stanislava Šaffová
Saint Elisabeth University of Health and Social Work, Bratislava, Slovak Republic

*Address all correspondence to: lanociar@r3.roburnet.sk

References

[1] Mustonen A, Alakokkare A-E, Salom C, et al. Age of first alcohol intoxication and psychiatric disorders in young adulthood – A prospective birth cohort study. Addictive Behaviors. 2021; **118**:106910

[2] Härkönen J, Mäkelä P. Elaborating the association of age at first drink with risky drinking: Results from a cross-sectional survey. Drugs: Education, Prevention and Policy. 24 Jul 2021:1-8. DOI: 10.1080/09687637.2021.1952932

[3] Newton-Howes G, Cook S, Martin G, Foulds JA, Boden JM. Comparison of age of first drink and age of first intoxication as predictors of substance use and mental health problems in adulthood. Drug and Alcohol Dependence. 2019; **194**:238-243

[4] Kraus L et al. "Are the times A-Changin"? Trends in adolescent substance use In Europe. Addiction. 2018;**113**:1317-1332

[5] Nociar A, Sierosławski J, Csémy L. Substance use among European students: East–west comparison between 1995 and 2011. Central European Journal of Public Health. 2016;**24**:281-288

[6] Radliff KM, Wheaton JE, Robinson K, Morris J. Illuminating the relationship between bullying and substance use among middle and high school youth. Addictive Behaviors. 2012;**37**:569-572

[7] Durand V, Hennessey J, Wells DS, Crothers LM, Kolbert JB, et al. Bullying and substance use in children and adolescents. Journal of Addiction Research and Therapy. 2013;**4**(4):58. DOI: 10.4172/2155-6105.1000 158

[8] Nociar A. Age, gender and substance use in relation to violence at primary and secondary schools in Slovakia. In: 4th World Conference: Violence in School and Public Policies. Abstracts. Lisbon: Calouste Gulbenkian Foundation; June 23-25, 2008. p. 100

[9] Zeigarnikova BV, Bratus BS. Očerki po Psichologii anomaľnogo Razvitija ličnosti. [Outlines of Psychology of Abnormal Development of Personality]. Moskva: Izd-vo. Moskovskogo Universiteta; 1980

[10] Novotný I, Nociar A. School without alcohol, tobacco and drugs: Prevention project and target population survey in Slovakia. In: Proceedings of the 38th and 21st International Institutes on the Prevention and Treatment of Alcoholism and Drug Dependence. Abstracts. Prague: ICAA, CIPAT; June 5-10, 1994. p. 180

[11] Olweus D. Bullying at School: What we Know and What we Can Do. Oxford: Blackwell Publishing; 2005. p. 140

[12] Skinner HA, Allen BA. Alcohol dependence syndrome: Measurement and validation. Journal of Abnormal Psychology. 1982;**91**:199-209

[13] Nociar A, Juráš L, Škultétyová M. Škála alkoholovej závislosti – ADS [Alcohol Dependence Scale – ADS]. Bratislava: Psychodiagnostické a didaktické testy, š.p; 1990. p. 51

[14] Nociar A. Záverečná správa z Prieskumu TAD u žiakov ZŠ, študentov SŠ a Ich učiteľov v Roku 2018 [Final Report from TAD Surveys among Elementary School Pupils, Secondary School Students and their Teachers in 2018]. Bratislava: VUDPaP; 2018. p. 87

[15] Nociar A. Európsky školský prieskum o alkohole a iných drogách

(ESPAD) v SR za rok 2019. In: Záverečná správa. [European School Survey on Alcohol and Other Drugs (ESPAD) in Slovakia in 2019. Final Report]. Bratislava: Research Institute for Child Psychology and Pathopsychology; 2019. p. 88

[16] Molinaro S, Vincente J, Benedetti E, Cerrai S, et al. ESPAD Report 2019: Results from the European School Survey Project on Alcohol and Other Drugs. Luxembourg: Publication Office of the European Union; 2020. p. 130

[17] Legleye S, Guignard R, Richard JB, Kraus L, Pabst A, Beck F. Properties of the cannabis abuse screening test (CAST) in the general population. International Journal of Methods in Psychiatric Research. 2015;**24**:170-183

[18] Kokkevi A, Gabhainn SN, Spyropoulou M. Early initiation of cannabis use: A cross-national European perspective. Journal of Adolescent Health. 2006;**39**:712-719

[19] Šátor B. Prvá Ponuka Alkoholu Od dospelého Vo vzťahu k začiatku fajčenia Marihuany [the First Offer of Alcohol by an Adult Related to the Beginning of Marihuana Smoking] [Thesis]. Bratislava: Saint Elisabeth University of Health and Social Work, Department of Psychology; 2021

Chapter 7

Screening and Brief Intervention in Substance Use Disorders: Its Clinical Utility and Feasibility Update from Available Literatures

Sambhu Prasad and Sweta Gupta

Abstract

It is found that substance use and related complications extend from occasional mild risky/harmful/hazardous use to severe conditions. The screening instruments may help to identify them in the initial state. The brief intervention (BI) is to bring change in unhealthy or risky substance use. The intervention is carried out by a vast array of trained professionals in various settings and it is valid across substances, age and ethno-culture groups. It has six common elements summarized by the acronym FRAMES (Feedback, Responsibility, Advise, Menu for change, Empathy and enhancing Self-efficacy). The BI has shown significant evidence of efficacy reducing substances and their harmful consequences with improving functionality and quality of life.

Keywords: screening tools, readiness to change, motivation, brief intervention

1. Introduction

Substance use disorders have become matters of global concern because of their impact on individual health, family dynamics, social consequences and criminal and legal problems. Broadly, substances can be classified based on their legal statuses as licit like alcohol, tobacco or illicit like opioids, cannabis, amphetamine and cocaine. World Drug Report (2022) say around 284 million people (aged 15–64) used drug in 2020 with a rise of 26% over the previous decade [1]. Globally around 2.3 billion people aged 15 and above are drinking alcohol [2]. Globally, approximately 39 deaths/100,000 populations are attributable to alcohol and illicit drug use (35 deaths to alcohol use, and 4 deaths to illicit drug use). The use of alcohol and illicit drugs accounts for almost 13 disability adjusted life years (DALYs) lost per 1000 population worldwide [3]. According to WHO, worldwide 3.3 million deaths every year result from harmful use of alcohol representing 5.9% of all deaths and 5.1% of the global burden of disease is attributable to alcohol consumption [2]. WHO research teams indicate that in South East Asia countries, one-third to one-fourth of male population drink alcohol with increasing trends among women [2]. The harmful use of alcohol causes huge health problems and social and economic burdens in societies. The harmful use of alcohol is a causal factor in more than 200 disease and injury conditions. Worldwide, 3 million deaths every year result from the harmful use of alcohol. This represents 5.3% of all deaths [4]. Alcohol use and cigarette smoking are rising rapidly in some of the developing regions [5]. Major increases in injecting drug use (opiate and amphetamine injection), which carries the highest health risks, were recorded in many regions of eastern European countries and South-East. Continuous tobacco use in any form may result in several cancer and data says that more than 8 million people die from tobacco use [6].

The use of cannabis is by far the most prevalent illicit substance used worldwide, next to the two licit substances tobacco and alcohol [1]. The effects of cannabis on mental health are multiple: multiple studies are available regarding cannabis and schizophrenia, cannabis and transient psychosis, affective disorders, panic, anxiety and amotivational syndrome [7]. The recently conducted largest national-level epidemiological study in India demonstrated that the prevalence figures of use of alcohol, cannabis and other illicit substances in males and females were 27.3 and 1.6, 5 and 0.6, and 4 and 0.2, respectively [8]. In India, the estimated numbers of alcohol users in 2005 were 62.5 million and among them, 10.6 million were dependent users. It has also revealed that 20–30% of all hospital admissions were due to alcohol-related problems [9]. Government statistics show only 21% of adult men and around 2% of women drink. But up to a fifth of this group, that is about 14 million people are dependent drinkers requiring 'help' [10]. It also reports that the percentage of drinking population aged under 21 years has increased from 2% to more than 14% in the past 15 years. The National Family Health Survey (NFHS) found changing trends between NFHS 2 (1998–1999) and NFHS 3 (2005–2006) reflecting an increase in alcohol use among males since NFHS 2, and an increase in tobacco use among women [11]. Tobacco use prevalence in India was high as 55.8% among male with maximum use in the age group 41–50 years. It is considered the primary licit substance of abuse in our country [8]. Studies on "bidi" smoking, the most common form of tobacco smoking in India, provide evidence towards causality of it as a carcinogenic substance [12]. Thus psychoactive substance use continues to take a significant toll, with valuable human lives and productive years of many persons being lost. Routine screening for substance use disorders could alter this statistic and get more people the help they need.

1.1 Workplace issues

In the National Survey on Drug Use and Health (United State) 22.4 million illicit drug users (68.9% aged 18 and above) are employed fully or partially. In the same survey, it was found that most binge drinkers and heavy alcohol users were also employed [79.3% (41.2 million) and 76.1% (12.4 million) respectively] [13].

Substance Abuse and Mental Health Services Administration report that 67.9% of the adult population of illegal drug users employed full-time or part-time indulged in binge and heavy alcohol use [14]. Studies show that when compared with non-substance users, substance-using employees are more likely to be: [15] less productive, up to 40% of accidents at work involve or are related to alcohol use, absenteeism is two to three times higher among habitual substance users, change jobs frequently and file a 'workers' compensation claim.

Many problems are encountered at workplace due to the substance use pattern of the worker. Workers under the influence of psychoactive substances are more likely to commit unsafe acts that cause damage to their own life, others' lives and the organization. There are safety risks from intoxication, negligence and impaired judgment. Problems with co-workers through increased workload on the non-substance user, disputes, grievances, intimidation and violence are common problems associated with substance use at the workplace. In India, a study was conducted among male industrial workers from Goa, which showed that 21% had hazardous levels of alcohol consumption [16]. Such levels of alcohol consumption were significantly associated with head injuries and hospitalization. The Central Sector Scheme of Assistance for prevention of Alcoholism and Substance (drugs) abuse and for Social Defence Services, Ministry of Social Justice and Empowerment, Government of India highlighted the need for interventions at the workplace. It encourages programs for prevention of alcoholism and drug abuse in the workplace. It provides financial assistance up to 25% of the expenditure for the setting up of a 15-bedded or 30-bedded Integrated Rehabilitation Centre for Addicts (IRCA) to the industry/enterprise having strength of at least 500 workers or more in a particular area [17].

1.2 Harmful substance use and screening

Screening aims to detect health problems or risk factors at an early stage before they have caused serious disease or other problems and is part of maintaining prevention practice activities in health care settings. Thus screening may be useful not only in the case of dependent but also for non-dependent users such as harmful or hazardous use [18, 19]. The limitations of using existing screening tests in primary care settings have been outlined, which are less useful for detecting harmful or hazardous use in non-dependent persons [20–22]. A large number of tools have been developed for identifying hazardous or harmful substance use. CAGE is a four-item validated questionnaire for identifying individuals with alcohol problems [23]. The Alcohol Use Disorders Identification Test (AUDIT) [24] is a screening tool for the identification of hazardous and harmful drinkers while the Fast Alcohol Screening Test (FAST) [25] is an abbreviated version of the AUDIT. There are many studies reporting success of AUDIT as screening and brief intervention (BI) in reducing alcohol-related problems in primary health care (PHC) settings [26]. However, it does not screen for other substances and related problems. This led to the development of ASSIST (Alcohol, Smoking and Substance Involvement Screening Test) [27].

1.3 Alcohol, Smoking and Substance Involvement Screening Test

WHO developed ASSIST as a simple scale for rapid screening of substance users to stratify them into three levels of risk severity (low, moderate and high risk) [27]. It is the first international screening test and an 8-item questionnaire that covers the use of all psychoactive substances and associated problems over the last 3 months. WHO-ASSIST was developed by an international group of addiction researchers and clinicians in response to the overwhelming public health burden associated with psychoactive substance use worldwide. The ASSIST has undergone significant testing in three sequential phases (I, II and III) to ensure that it is a feasible, reliable, valid, flexible, comprehensive and cross-culturally relevant tool. ASSIST is currently in its fourth phase aimed at worldwide dissemination. It helps in early identification of substance use-related health risks and substance use disorders in PHS, general medical care and other settings. Gryczynski et al. [28] did a study on validation and performance of ASSIST among adolescent primary care patients as it has only been validated with adults and concluded that it is a promising as a research and screening/brief assessment tool with adolescents, but revisions to clinical risk thresholds are warranted. In another study, in Mexico, to determine the psychometric properties of the self-administered ASSIST test in university undergraduate students (n = 1176), the authors concluded that it is a valid screening instrument to identify at-risk cases due to substance use in this population [29]. Silva et al., did an integrative review including 26 articles to systematize the knowledge and the learning of how the instrument ASSIST has been applied. They concluded that ASSIST focused on helping the identification and classification of psychoactive substance use and highlighted its importance in screening the involvement with alcohol and other drugs and is effective in PHC [30].

1.4 Brief interventions for harmful substance use

BI is a treatment strategy structured in nature, short duration (around 5–30 minutes) offered with the aim to assist an individual to cease or reduce the use of psychoactive substances [31]. It generally aims to moderate a person's substance consumption to sensible levels and to eliminate harmful drinking practices rather than to insist on complete abstinence from drinking—although abstinence may be encouraged, if appropriate. Brief interventions typically consist of one to four short counselling sessions with a trained interventionist (e.g., physician, psychologist and social worker) [31]. The specific stages of change include Pre-contemplation (not thinking about changing), Contemplation (thinking about change, weighing up the pros and cons and information/resource gathering) and Action (actually cutting down or stopping) [32]. But the technique of FRAMES (feedback, responsibility, advice, menu, empathy, self-efficacy) and motivational interviewing has been used in a large number of studies to facilitate a change in the behaviour [33, 34].

1.5 ASSIST-linked brief intervention for harmful substance use

While it is clear that brief interventions are effective in substance use, it appears that implementation within health settings may be hindered by a number of barriers. These include lack of time, lack of staff, knowledge and skills to conduct the screening and intervention [31]. To combat these identified limitations, ASSIST-linked BI was developed by the WHO [35]. It is a short but structured and less time-consuming intervention. It is linked to the score from the ASSIST screening questionnaire via the use of the ASSIST feedback report card, which records the participants' ASSIST scores and presents the risks associated with the participants' current pattern of substance use. Then a discussion to commence BI with the client in a non-confrontational way to change their substance use as per ASSIST score (moderate or high risk group). The ASSIST-linked BI is a short intervention lasting 5–15 minutes given to clients. It is a simple, less time-consuming, step-by-step approach to motivate clients to reduce their substance use and produces very little resistance or client defensiveness. It is based on components of BI from the FRAMES model and motivational interviewing [33, 34].

2. Review of literature

2.1 Screening and brief intervention in workplace settings

The workplace is an ideal setting for alcohol and drug user for health prevention and interventions as most of them are employed and spend a lot of time there [36, 37]. Jenkins [38] in 1986 showed that there was a strong correlation between drinking and absence from work in a study of young civil service staff in Britain. In a study from Australia, workplace can be an effective setting to reduce substance-related problems [39]. Hermansson et al. [40], demonstrated the feasibility of screening and delivering a BI at the workplace in Sweden within a routine health check of employees conducted by the occupational health service. Studies show that regular occupational health check-up with screening the substance use at regular intervals is quite effective in early interventions [41, 42]. In the study conducted by Richmond et al. [43], found a significant reduction in the number of drinks consumed by the women in the intervention group in a matched group comparison. Watson et al. [44], found that there was scope within the workplace to promote initiatives in relation to reducing hazardous and harmful levels of alcohol consumption, which was cost-effectiveness, amenable to an assessment of lifestyle issues and promoting health and wellbeing. Hermansson et al. investigated the results of screening and BI in a large transport company (including 990 employees, mainly men, have found that 20% of those screened were drinking hazardously). The results at 12 months showed that the interventions were effective but screening itself acted positively in terms of reducing drinking [45]. The study conducted by Zibe-Piegel and Boerngen-Lacerda [46] recommended the routine practice of screening and BI in the workplace as it was found to be feasible and helpful in earlier detection and referral to treatment services for harmful substance use. Ito et al., conducted RCT on BI at the workplace for heavy drinkers among industrial workers in Japan. The alcohol-free days in the BI group significantly increased by 93.0% at 12 months. The authors concluded that BI at the workplace was effective in increasing the number of alcohol-free days. However, the effectiveness of decreasing alcohol consumption was unclear, which could be explained by alcohol screening itself causing a reduction in drinking [47].

2.2 Effectiveness of brief interventions in reducing alcohol use—meta analysis and systematic reviews

Convincing evidence exists about the effectiveness of BI for harmful alcohol users admitted to general hospital wards and in PHC settings. Wilk et al., studied 12 RTCs in which BI was given to heavy drinkers and found that heavy drinkers in the interventional group were twice as likely to moderate their drinking pattern after 6–12 months compared to the controlled group [48]. Ballesteros et al., did a study on efficacy of BIs on hazardous drinkers and included 13 studies. There was no clear evidence of a dose-effect relationship. Although indicating smaller effect sizes than previous meta-analyses, it does support the moderate efficacy of BIs [49]. Bertholet et al. [50], had a study on reduction of alcohol consumption by a brief intervention, which included 19 trials of 5639 individuals and it was found that that brief alcohol intervention was effective in reducing alcohol consumption at 6 and 12 months. McQueen et al. [51], did study on BIs for heavy alcohol users admitted to general hospital wards, which included 14 studies involving 4041 male participants and it was concluded that patients receiving BIs had a greater reduction in alcohol consumption compared to those in control groups at 6 and 9 months follow up, but it was not maintained at 1 year and had significantly fewer deaths. Sullivan et al. [52], did a study on meta-analysis of the efficacy of non-physician BIs for unhealthy alcohol use: implications for the patient-centred medical home including 13 studies and showed 1.7 times fewer standard drinks per week than control conditions. A meta-analysis on the effects on mortality of BIs for problem drinking concluded that brief interventions may reduce mortality rates among problem drinkers by an estimated 23–26% [53].

2.3 BI and alcohol consumption in primary health care settings

There is substantial evidence of the benefits of screening and BI for alcohol problems in PHC settings. BI was found to be effective at PHC setting in reduction of alcohol consumption and it is cost-effectively related to various problems associated with substance use [54–56]. Moreover, BIs have been found to be effective in both primary and secondary care settings for hazardous or harmful alcohol use when delivered under research conditions [57, 58]. Brief interventions have been shown to be cost-effective for hazardous drinkers whose alcohol use put them at risk of alcohol-related problems, but who have few symptoms of alcohol dependence [24, 59]. Brief interventions have been used to encourage those with more serious dependence to engage or improve compliance with more intensive treatment [60]. Lock et al., had conducted a study on cluster RCT to test the effectiveness and cost-effectiveness of screening and BI for patients in PHC in which the intervention group was given 5–10-minute BI and standard advice was offered in the control group. However, ANOVA revealed no statistically significant difference between intervention and control patients at follow-up in alcohol use and economic benefits [61]. Chang et al., conducted an RCT to test the effectiveness of BI and the involvement of their partners in the PHC setting using T-ACE as screening tool and assessed the outcome measures in women with alcohol use, alcohol abstinence self-efficacy score andpartners' collateral report on the subjects' alcohol use. The intervention group received a 25-minute BI by either a nurse or doctor and the control group as usual care. It was found that alcohol use declined in both groups and BI was more effective in women group [62]. Ockene et al., made a study to compare the efficacy of BI in PHC setting with the control group. A 5–10 minutes patient-centred BI found significant reductions in alcohol consumption [63]. Similarly, Goodall et al. [64], reported that two brief sessions in the intervention group showed significantly greater reductions in the frequency of alcohol use variables.

In a community-based study in North India, a sample was followed for 3 months in which 90 male subjects (20–45 years) with an AUDIT score between 8 and 24 consented to participate and were allocated alternatively to the BI or simple advice (SA) protocols. The study showed significant differences across interventions, with a decrease in severity of dependence in the last 30 days, composite ASI (Addiction Severity Index) scores and improvement in physical and psychological quality of life. However, the result was not sustained for a longer duration and the author claimed that booster sessions were needed [65].

2.4 BI and Substance use in various settings

Gryczynski et al., assessed the effectiveness of BI at 6-month follow-up at a rural health care centre. The screening was done with AUDIT and yes/no questions about past year's use of any illegal drug. Outcome measures were recorded as changes in self-reported frequency of illicit drug use, alcohol use and alcohol intoxication. Study showed that there was a greater magnitude of change in drinking behaviours and reductions in illicit drug use. While substantial, it did not differ significantly based on service variables [66]. Bertha et al., conducted a study in which screening, brief interventions and referral to treatment (SBIRT) were used in a wide variety of medical settings. The screening was done with AUDIT and Drug Abuse Screening Test (DAST) and compared illicit drug use at intake and 6 months after drug screening and interventions. Study has shown that the intervention was feasible to implement, and the self-reported status at 6 months indicated significant improvements over baseline for illicit drug use and heavy alcohol use and also in functional domains [67]. Mitchell et al., had done pre–post analysis to assess the effectiveness of screening, brief interventions and referral to treatment (SBIRT) at 6-month follow-up at a school-based program. The screening was done with CRAFFT. It examined the outcomes of SBIRT services and compared the extent of change in substance use based on the intensity of intervention received. Participants receiving any intervention reported significant reductions in frequency of drinking to intoxication ($p < 0.05$) and drug use ($p < 0.001$) [68]. In another study done by Beintrein et al., in whichan RCT was conducted in inner-city teaching hospital outpatient clinics. Interventional group was given a brief motivational intervention and compared with the control group at 3 and 6 months follow-up. The intervention group was more likely to be abstinent than the control group for cocaine as well as heroin use with a reduction of cocaine level in the hair [69]. Similarly, Saunders et al. [70], also found that BI delivered to opiate users attending a methadone program to be effective in increasing participants' compliance with treatment and motivation to quit drug use, as well as reducing the number of reported drug-related problems and rate of relapse. Although there is growing evidence in support of BIs for a range of illicit substances, some studies have failed to find significant effects [71]. In a systematic review done by Young et al., on effectiveness of brief interventions as part of the SBIRT model for reducing the nonmedical use of psychoactive substances that identified 8836 records. They concluded that insufficient evidence exists as to whether BIs, as part of SBIRT, were effective or ineffective for reducing the use of substance and harm related to it [72].

Cannabis users generally had a low level of motivation to quit its use and have a concern about stigma to assess the treatment [73]. Despite all these the BIs have recently been developed for cannabis use in an attempt to address the gaps in treatment engagement, and a small number of studies have been conducted with promising results [74–77].

Stephens et al., in their first RCT, found two 90-minute individual sessions (comprising assessment, personalised feedback and advice) to be as effective as more extensive treatment and more effective than no treatment in reducing cannabis use and related problems [78]. Similarly, Walker et al., also found two sessions of motivational enhancement therapy delivered to adolescent cannabis users resulted in reduced cannabis use and fewer negative consequences at 12 months compared to a delayed-treatment control group [79].

In a simple single-group pre–post design, Denering and Spear [80] found screening and a brief 10–15 minute intervention delivered to college students resulted in reductions in the proportion of students reporting cannabis use at 6 months.

BIs for smoking cessation have also been found to be highly effective. A systematic review by Stead et al. [81], (included 42 clinical trials) conducted since 1972 found that brief advice to patients to quit smoking increased the likelihood of a cessation attempt, as well as abstinence at the 12-month follow-up with an additional benefit of more intensive advice on quit rates.

2.5 The ASSIST-linked brief intervention

Spear et al. [82], did a study on substance abuse screening and BI in a mental health clinic and concluded that administration of the ASSIST in a campus mental health clinic was feasible and brought an opportunity for discussion related to substance use. Humeniuk et al., did an international RCT to evaluate the effectiveness of ASSIST-linked BI for illicit drugs (cannabis, cocaine, ATS and opioids). Participants were recruited from PHC settings in four countries (Australia, Brazil, India and the United States of America) and were randomly allocated to an intervention or waitlist control group at baseline and the groups were followed up after 3 months. A total of 731 participants were recruited from a variety of PHC settings for the international study (Australia n = 171; Brazil n = 165; India n = 177 and United States of America n = 218). Participants were aged between 16 and 62 years. It was concluded that the ASSIST-linked BI was effective in getting participants to reduce their substance use and risk as supported by feedback from at 3 months follow-up [83]. Zibe-Piegel and Boerngen-Lacerda did research work from city hall in a southern city of Brazil representative sample of employees (n = 1310), 144 individuals in risky use and 139 dependents on tobacco, alcohol and/or other substances where ASSIST-linked BI was used during 3-month follow-up. It showed a significant reduction in ASSIST scores and was feasible in workplace to prevent hazardous/ harmful substance use without prejudice or stigma, enabling earlier detection, intervention and treatment referral [46]. Assanangkornchai et al., demonstrated the implementation, acceptability and uptake of the screening and BI program based on the ASSIST to help decrease substance misuse in primary care in Thailand. Here 5931 patients were screened with the ASSIST. Of these, 29.6% and 3.4% were in the moderate and high-risk groups, respectively and were offered BI or other treatments. The ASSIST detected many substance users capable of benefiting from the intervention. The program was well received by patients and staff and suggested as a model for introducing similar procedures into developing countries [84]. Saitz et al., did a study to test the efficacy of two brief counselling interventions for unhealthy drug use (any illicit drug use or prescription drug misuse). A total of 528 adult primary care patients were randomised into three groups after screening with ASSIST scores greater than or equal to 4. A brief negotiated interview (10- to 15-minute structured interviews) and an adaptation of motivational interviewing (30- to 45-minute intervention based on motivational interviewing with a 20- to 30-minute booster) and compared with no brief intervention. There were no significant effects of brief negotiated interviews or an adaptation of motivational interviewing on self-reported measures of drug use and its consequences. These results did not support widespread implementation of illicit drug use and prescription drug misuse screening and brief intervention [85]. Loretta et al., provided preliminary evidence of the effectiveness of ASSIST-linked BI in a college mental health clinic where 453 students (ages 18–24) participated in the evaluation and completed baseline and 6-month follow-up interviews. Study showed a slight reduction in the rates and number of days (in the prior 30 days) of binge drinking and marijuana use and it was concluded that routine screening and BI procedures in a mental health setting may reduce problematic substance use among college students [86]. Pengpid et al., did RCT including screening and concurrent BI of conjoint hazardous or harmful alcohol and tobacco use in hospital outpatients in Thailand. Results of the interaction (group × time) effects indicated that there were statistically significant differences between the three study groups [tobacco only intervention, alcohol only intervention and the polydrug use (alcohol and tobacco) integrated intervention groups] over the 6-month follow-up on the ASSIST tobacco score and past week tobacco use abstinence. The result show reduction in scores in all six outcome parameters (Alcohol ASSIST score, low alcohol risk score, past week tobacco abstinence or low alcohol risk score and past week tobacco abstinence and low alcohol risk score) [87]. Lasebikan and Ola did a study to determine whether screening, BI and referral for treatment (RT) can reduce the prevalence of tobacco use in rural and semi-rural settings in Nigeria. Participants received a single ASSIST-linked BI and RT at entry, and a booster ASSIST BI and RT at 3 months. It shows that BI with booster sessions at 3 months had a significant effect on tobacco use in people living in community and suggested the need for promotion of such program [88].

2.6 The ASSIST-linked brief intervention at the workplace

There are few published international studies about the implementation of a screening-linked BI using WHO's ASSIST screening scale in the workplace settings. There is a single published study from India conducted by Joseph et al. [89], on the feasibility of conducting the ASSIST-linked screening and BI from a tertiary hospital in north India (from this same institute). The study showed that it was feasible to use ASSIST for screening at the workplace to identify risk level substance use and to use ASSIST-BI for their brief intervention [90]. Joseph et al. [90], also studied the effect of ASSIST-linked BI and compared the mean pre and post-alcohol ASSIST scores in workplace settings for harmful drinking among class C employees of a tertiary hospital in north India. A sample of 39 workers with moderate and high-risk levels of alcohol use was identified by randomly screening 162 employees with ASSIST. Employees who were identified as moderate and high-risk drinkers by the ASSIST were given the BI as per WHO ASSIST-linked BI [90].A significant difference over 4 months ($p < 0.001$) was noticed where the mean ASSIST score reduced from 26.55 (pre-intervention) to 20.06 (post-intervention). There were also improvements in other variables like alcohol consumption, strong desire to use alcohol and health, social and legal problems due

ASSIST score	Group	Baseline		3-Month follow up		*F* value	*p*-Value	Power
		Mean	SD	Mean	SD			
Tobacco	Control	28.46	2.42	26.62	2.57	104.34	<0.001	100%
	Intervention	29.35	2.82	19.29	3.26			
	Interaction effect					218.95	<0.001	100%
	Main effect					31.40	<0.001	100%
Alcohol	Control	31.18	4.49	27.66	4.03	246.16	<0.001	100%
	Intervention	32.75	2.72	11.62	5.87			
	Interaction effect					482.06	<0.001	100%
	Main effect					48.03	<0.001	100%
Cannabis	Control	33.40	2.07	26.40	1.94	25.11	<0.001	99.3%
	Intervention	31.66	5.42	9.50	3.83			
	Interaction effect					92.87	<0.001	100%
	Main effect					30.26	<0.001	99.8%

ASSIST: Alcohol, Smoking and Substance Involvement Screening Test. Bonferroni correction is done to counteract the problem of multiple comparisons. Adjusted alpha (α) = α/k (number of comparison). (0.05/3 = 0.016).

Table 1.
Comparison of groups at baseline and follow-up on the basis of ASSIST using two-way repeated measure ANOVA.

Substance	Control (N = 34) Mean and SD	Intervention (N = 33) Mean and SD	(t-Value/U = Mann Whitney/$\chi 2$ = Chi square) p-value
Tobacco			
ASSIST score	28.32 (±2.38) Range [22–31]	29.27 (±2.75) Range [22–36]	(t = −1.181) p = 0.242
Risk level	Moderate (n = 7) Severe (n = 27)	Moderate (n = 4) Severe (n = 29)	($\chi 2$ = 0.875) p = 0.350
Alcohol			
ASSIST score	31.20 (±3.4) Range [24–38]	32.67 (±2.65) [26–37]	(t =−1.610) p = 0.113
Risk level	Moderate (n = 4) High (n = 26)	Moderate (n = 1) Severe (n = 30)	($\chi 2$ = 2.070) p = 0.150
Cannabis			
ASSIST score	32.83 (±2.31) Range [30–35]	31.85 (±4.98) Range [22–37]	(t = 0.120) p = 0.639
Risk level	Moderate (n = 0) High (n = 6)	Moderate (n = 1) High (n = 6)	($\chi 2$ = 1.091) p = 0.296

Risky use of substances was assessed with an application of ASSIST and thus subjects were categorised into different risk levels on the pattern of substance use. As per Table 2, the mean ASSIST score of tobacco users at baseline in the control group was 28.32 (±2.38) and ranged between 22 and 31. Most of the subjects were at high levels of risky use of tobacco (high level, n = 27 and moderate level, n = 3). In the intervention group, the mean ASSIST score was 29.27 (±2.75) and ranged between 22 and 36. Most of the subjects were at high levels of risky use of tobacco (high level, n = 29 and moderate level, n = 4). However, both the groups did not differ statistically on basis of ASSIST score and severity (p = 0.242), (p = 0.350), respectively.
In the same Table 2, the mean ASSIST score of alcohol users at baseline in the control group was 31.20 (±−3.4) and ranged between 24 and 38. Most of the subjects were at high levels of risky use of alcohol (high level, n = 26 and moderate level, n = 4]. In the intervention group, the mean ASSIST score was 32.67 (±2.65) and ranged between 26 and 37. Most of the subjects were at high levels of risky use of alcohol [high level, n = 30 and moderate level, n = 1]. However, both the groups did not differ statistically on basis of ASSIST score and risk level (p = 0.113), (p = 0.150), respectively.
In the same Table 2, the mean ASSIST score of cannabis users at baseline in the control group was 32.83 (±2.31) and ranged between 30 and 35. All the cannabis users were at high levels of risky use (high level, n = 6 and moderate level, n = 0). In the intervention group, the mean ASSIST score was 31.85 (±4.98) and ranged between 22 and 37. Here also most of the subjects were at high levels of risky use of cannabis (high level, n = 6 and moderate level, n = 1). However, both the groups did not differ statistically on basis of ASSIST score and risk level (p = 0.639), (p = 0.296), respectively.

Table 2.
ASSIST score and risk level of randomised groups at baseline.

to alcohol at follow-up (p < 0.001) [90]. In a recent study using randomised controlled trial design, to study the efficacy of ASSIST-linked BI where major objectives were to reduce risky substance use among class C male workers, enhance the progress of subjects through the stages of change and motivate the subjects to seek treatment [91]. The inferential analysis showed that participants receiving BI had a significant reduction of ASSIST scores for all risky use of substances compared with Control. Thus there was a significant reduction in the risk level of all categories of substance use in the intervention group compared with the control group.

The interaction effects in the stage of change indicate that the participants in the intervention group who were using tobacco had significantly changed their stage to action stage more than that of the control group. Similar significant changes were also noticed in the risky alcohol users of the intervention group compared with that of the control group. However, in the risky users of cannabis, the interaction effects indicate that there was no significant change in the contemplation stage in both groups but significant changes were noticed in precontemplation and action stages in the intervention group compared with the control group.

The interaction effect on quality of life shows that the participants receiving BI had significantly increased scores for all the domains of WHOQOL-BREF compared with that of the control group. Participants receiving BI were significantly more motivated to seek treatment compared to the control group.

2.7 Effect of the ASSIST BI on specific substance involvement score

Two-way repeated measures ANOVA results show that there was a significant reduction of mean tobacco ASSIST scores over time among groups ($F = 218.95$, $p < 0.001$ and observed power 100%). There was also a significant reduction in mean scores among the groups. Moreover, there was a significant interaction effect and the

Substance	Control ($N = 32$)	Intervention ($N = 31$)	(t-Value/$\chi2$ = Chi square) p-value
	Mean and SD	**Mean and SD**	
Tobacco use			
ASSIST score	26.62 (±2.57) Range [22–31]	19.29 (±3.26) Range [11–25]	($t = 9.913$) $p < 0.001$
Risk level	Moderate ($n = 9$) High ($n = 23$)	Moderate ($n = 31$) High ($n = 0$)	($\chi2 = 35.093$) $p < 0.001$
Alcohol use			
ASSIST score	27.66 (±4.03) Range [24–38]	11.62 (±5.87) [5–24]	($t = 11.831$) $p < 0.001$
Risk level	Low ($n = 0$) Moderate ($n = 8$) High ($n = 19$)	Low ($n = 17$) Moderate ($n = 12$) High ($n = 0$)	($\chi2 = 36.775$) $p < 0.001$
Cannabis use			
ASSIST score	26.40 (±1.94) Range [23–28]	9.52 (±3.83) Range [5–21]	($t = 8.805$) $p < 0.001$
Risk level	Moderate ($n = 2$) High ($n = 3$)	Moderate ($n = 6$) High ($n = 0$)	($\chi2 = 4.950$) $p = 0.026$

ASSIST score was re-assessed after 3 months of follow-up. The mean ASSIST score of tobacco in the control group was 26.62 (±2.57) and ranged between 22 and 31 whereas in the intervention group it was19.29 (±3.26) and it was statistically significant (t = 9.913; p < 0.001). It means that most of the subjects from the intervention group were at a moderate level and none were at high level of risky use of tobacco (moderate risk, n = 31 and high risk, n = 0), and it was statistically significant as compared with the control group (moderate, n = 9 and high level, n = 23) [χ2 = 35.093; p < 0.001] (Table 3).
The mean ASSIST score of alcohol users in the control group was 27.66 (±4.03) whereas in the intervention group was 11.62 (5.87) and it was statistically significant [t = 11.831; p < 0.001]. It means that most of the subjects from the intervention group were at low and moderate levels and none were at high level of risky alcohol use (moderate risk, n = 12 and low risk, n = 17), and it was statistically significant as compared to the control group (moderate, n = 8 and high level, n = 19) [χ2 = 36.775; p < 0.001] (Table 3).
Similarly, none of the subjects were at a high-risk level of cannabis use in the intervention group as compared with the control group. Further, there was a statistically significant difference in risky use of cannabis in the intervention group as compared with the control group with respect to the mean ASSIST score and mean risk level of cannabis used [(t = 8.805; p < 0.001), (χ2 = 4.950; p = 0.026)], respectively (Table 3).

Table 3.
ASSIST score and risk level of randomised groups at follow-up.

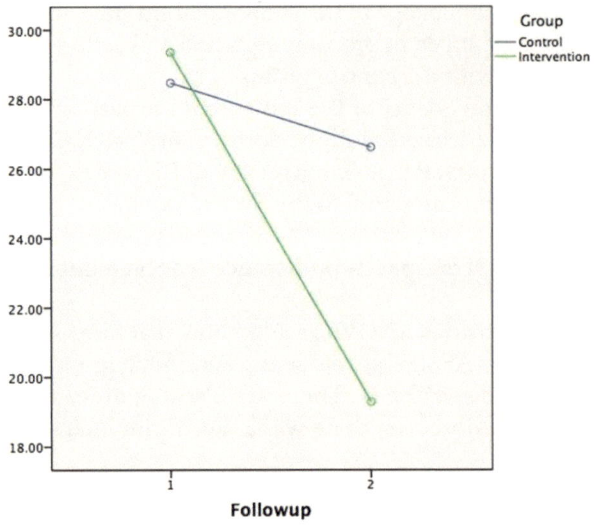

Figure 1.
Change in total ASSIST score for risky tobacco use.

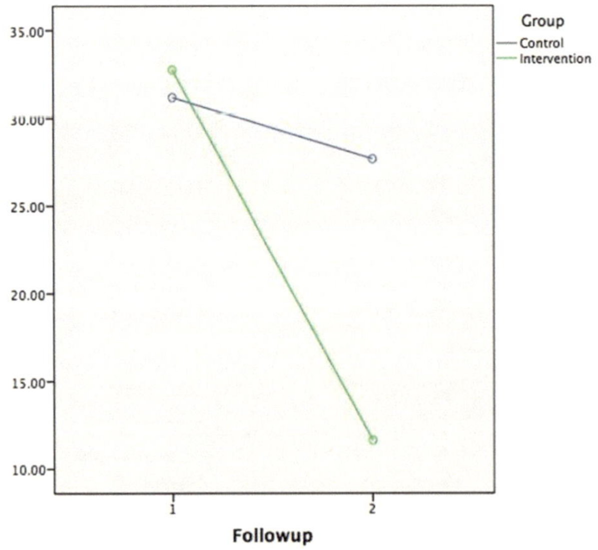

Figure 2.
Change in total ASSIST score for risky alcohol use.

group receiving the BI at baseline had significantly lower mean tobacco ASSIST scores at follow-up compared with the control group ($F = 104.34$, $p < 0.001$ and observed power 100%) (**Tables 1–3**). The result is shown graphically in **Figure 1**.

Similarly, statistical significance reduction of mean alcohol as well as cannabis ASSIST scores over time among the groups ($F = 482.06$, $p < 0.001$, observed power 100% and $F = 92.87$ $p = 0.001$, observed power 100%, respectively). There was also a significant reduction in mean scores among the groups using alcohol and cannabis. Moreover, there was a significant interaction effect and the group receiving the BI at baseline had significantly lower mean alcohol as well as cannabis ASSIST

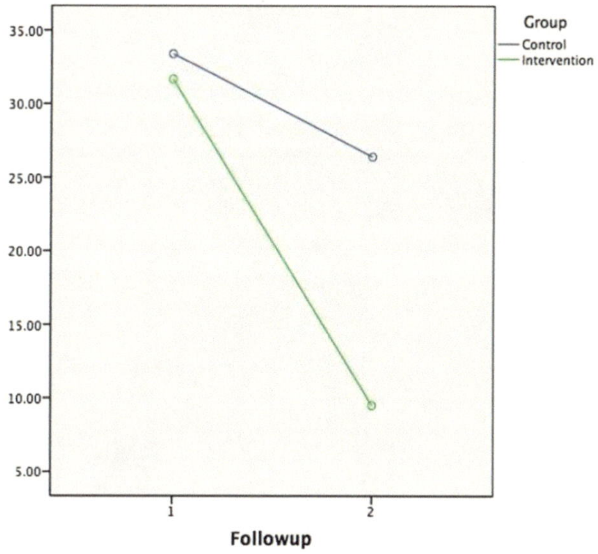

Figure 3.
Change in total ASSIST score for risky cannabis use.

scores ($F = 246.16$, $p < 0.001$, observed power 100% and $F = 25.11$, $p < 0.001$, observed power 99.3%, respectively) (**Tables 1–3**). Results are shown graphically in **Figures 2** and **3**.

3. Conclusion

BI has clear scientific principles in harm reduction, stage of change, motivational interview, simple to deliver and cost-effectiveness. It can use even in opportunistic setting by non-specialist professionals. It can be an extended service for an individual who needs help but not seeking treatment from specialised centres. Thus BI could be considered as part of clinician's responsibility, in addition as such prescribing medicine, ordering test, performing surgical procedures, filling medical forms, etc. It has favourable outcome as evidences show reduction and prevention of various substance-related consequences.

Author details

Sambhu Prasad[1*] and Sweta Gupta[2]

1 Department of Psychiatry, All India Institute of Medical Sciences (AIIMS) Patna, India

2 Department of Orthodontics, Patna Dental College and Hospital, Patna, India

*Address all correspondence to: sambhu3011@gmail.com

References

[1] United Nations Office on Drugs and Crime. World Drug Report 2016. [online] Availabe from: http://www.unodc.org/documents/wdr/WDR_2022/WRD2022_eng_web.pdf. [Accessed: 11 July 2022]

[2] Global status report on alcohol and health 2018. [online] Available from: http://www.Who.int [Accessed: 10 July 2022]

[3] Atlas on substance use. Resources for the prevention and treatment of substance use disorders. Geneva: World Health Organization; 2010. [online] Available from: http://www.who.int/substance_abuse/publications/treatment/en/. [Accessed: 10 June 2022]

[4] Global strategy to reduce harmful use of alcohol 2018. [online] Available from: http://www.whqlibdoc.who.int. [Accessed: 14 June 2022]

[5] Uchtenhagen A. Substance use problems in developing countries. Bulletin of the World Health Organization. 2004;**82**:461-468

[6] WHO report on the global tobacco epidemic 2021: addressing new and emerging products. Geneva: World Health Organization; 2021. Licence: CC BY-NC-SA 3.0 IGO [Accessed: 10 July 2022]

[7] Grover S, Basu D. Cannabis and psychopathology: update 2004. Indian Journal of Psychiatry. 2004;**46**:299-309

[8] Ambekar A, Agrawal A, Rao R, Mishra AK, Khandelwal SK, Chadda RK. on behalf of the group of investigators for the National Survey on Extent and Pattern of Substance Use in IndiaMagnitude of Substance Use in India. New Delhi: Ministry of Social Justice and Empowerment, Government of India; 2019. [Accessed: 11 July 2022]

[9] Gururaj G, Girish N, Benegal V, Chandra V, Pandav R. Public health problems caused by harmful use of alcohol – Gaining less or losing more? Alcohol Control series 2, World Health Organisation. New Delhi: Regional Office for South East Asia; 2006

[10] Prasad R. Alcohol use on the rise in India. The Lancet. 2009;**373**:17-18

[11] National Family Health Survey India. [online] Available from: http://www.nfhsindia.org/nfhs3.html. [Accessed: 10 June 2022]

[12] IARC Working Group on the Evaluation of Carcinogenic Risks to Humans. Tobacco smoke and involuntary smoking. IARC MonogrEvalCarcinog Risks Hum. 2004;**83**:1-1438

[13] National Survey on Drug Use and Health: Dress Rehearsal Final Report. Substance Abuse and Mental Health Services Administration 2013. [online] Available from: http://www.samhsa.gov/NSDUH-DressRehearsal-2013. [Accessed: 11 July 2012]

[14] Rockville MD. Results from the 2012 National Survey on Drug Use and Health: Summary of National Findings. Substance Abuse and Mental Health Services Administration, NSDUH Series H-46, HHS Publication No. (SMA) 13-4795: Substance Abuse and Mental Health Services Administration, 2013. [online] Available from: http://www.samhsa.gov/data/NSDUH/2012.html. [Accessed: 13 June 2022]

[15] Murthy P, editor. Partnerships for Drug Demand Reduction in

India: Developing Community Drug Rehabilitation and Workplace Prevention Programmes. United Nations Drug Control Programme, Ministry of Social Justice and Empowerment, Government of India, International Labour Organization, European Commission; 2002. [online] Available from: http://www.unodc.org/india/en/Partnerships_808_Report.html. [Accessed: 28 June 2022]

[16] Chagas M, Gaunekar G, Patel V, Kukalekar DS, Fernandes J. The prevalence and correlates of hazardous drinking in industrial workers: a study from Goa, India. Alcohol and Alcoholism. 2003;**38**:79-83

[17] The Central Sector Scheme of Assistance for prevention of Alcoholism and Substance (drugs) abuse and for Social Defence Services, Government of India Ministry of Social Justice and Empowerment January, 2015. [online] Available from: http://www.socialjustice.nic.in. [Accessed: 19 July 2022]

[18] Royal Australian College of General Practitioners. Putting prevention into practice. A guide for the implementation of prevention in the general practice setting. Melbourne, Australia: RACGP; 1998

[19] Royal Australian College of General Practitioners. Guidelines for Preventive Activities in General Practice. 2nd ed. Melbourne, Australia: RACGP; 2002

[20] Institute of Medicine Broadening. The Base of Treatment for Alcohol Problems. Washington DC: National Academic Press; 1990

[21] Skinner HA. Early detection of alcohol & drug problems-why? Australian Drug and Alcohol Review. 1987;**6**:293-301

[22] McPherson TL, Hersh RK. Brief substance use screening instruments for primary care settings: a review. Journal of Substance Abuse Treatment. 2000;**18**:193-202

[23] Erwing JA. Detecting alcoholism: the CAGE questionnaire. Journal of the American Medical Association. 1984;**252**:1905-1907

[24] Babor TF, Higgins-Biddle JC. Brief Intervention for Hazardous and Harmful Drinking: A Manual for Use in Primary Care. Geneva: World Health Organization, Department of Mental Health and Substance Dependence; 2001. [online] Available from: http://whqlibdoc.who.int/hq/2001/WHO_MSD_MSB_01.6b.pdf. [Accessed: 19 June 2022]

[25] Hodgson R, Alwyn T, John B, Thom B, Smith A. The FAST alcohol screening test. Alcohol and Alcoholism. 2001;**37**:61-66

[26] Saunders JB, Aasland OG, Babor TF, de la Fuente JR, Grant M. Development of the Alcohol Use Disorders Identification Test (AUDIT): WHO collaborative project on early detection of persons with harmful alcohol consumption II. Addiction. 1993;**88**:791-804

[27] WHO ASSIST Working Group. The Alcohol, Smoking and Substance Involvement Screening Test (ASSIST): Development, Reliability and Feasibility. Addiction. 2002;**97**:1183-1194

[28] Gryczynski J, Kelly SM, Mitchell SG, Kirk A, O'Grady KE, Schwartz RP. Validation and performance of the Alcohol, Smoking, and Substance Involvement Screening Test (ASSIST) among adolescent primary care patients. Addiction. 2015;**110**:240-247

[29] Sainz MT, Rosete-Mohedano MG, Rey GN, Vélez NAM, García SC, Cisneros DP. Validity and reliability of the Alcohol, Smoking, and Substance Involvement Screening Test (ASSIST) in University Students. Adicciones. 2016;**28**:19-27

[30] Silva AC, Lucchese R, Vargas LS, Benício PR, Vera I. Application of the Alcohol, Smoking and Substance Involvement Screening Test (ASSIST) instrument: an integrative review. Revista gaucha de enfermagem. 2016;**37**(1):e52918. [online] Available from: http://www.scielo.br/rgenf. Accessed: 11 July 2012

[31] Roche A, Freeman T. Brief interventions: good in theory but weak in practice. Drug and Alcohol Review. 2004;**23**:11-18

[32] Bien TH, Miller WR, Tonigan S. Brief interventions for alcohol problems: a review. Addiction. 1993;**88**:315-336

[33] Miller WR, Rollnick S. Motivational Interviewing: Preparing People for Change. 2nd ed. New York: The Guilford Press; 2002

[34] Prochaska JA, DiClemente CC. Transtheoretical therapy: towards a more integrative model of change. Psychotherapy. 1982;**19**:276-288

[35] Humeniuk RE, Dennington V, Ali RL. The Effectiveness of a Brief Intervention for Illicit Drugs Linked to the ASSIST Screening Test in Primary Health Care Settings: a Technical Report of Phase III Findings of the WHO ASSIST Randomised Controlled Trial. Geneva: World Health Organization; 2008

[36] Roman PM, Blum TC. The workplace and alcohol problem prevention. Alcohol Research & Health. 2002;**26**:49-57

[37] Hodgins DC, Williams R, Munro G. workplace responsibility, stress, alcohol availability and norms as predictors of alcohol consumption-related problems among employed workers. Substance Use & Misuse. 2009;**44**:2062-2069

[38] Jenkins R. Sex differences in alcohol consumption and its associated morbidity in young civil servants. British Journal of Addiction. 1986;**81**:525-535

[39] Pidd K, Roche AM, Buisman-Pijlman F. Intoxicated workers: findings from a national Australian survey. Addiction. 2011;**106**:1623-1633

[40] Hermansson U, Knutsson A, Ronberg S, Brandt L. Feasibility of brief intervention in the workplace for the detection and treatment of excessive alcohol consumption. International Journal of Occupational and Environmental Health. 1998;**4**:71-78

[41] Henderson MM, Davies JB, Hutcheson G. Alcohol in the Workplace. London: Department of Education and Employment; 1995

[42] Fauske S, Wilkinson DA, Shain M. Communicating alcohol and drug prevention strategies and models across cultural boundaries: preliminary report on an ILO/WHO/UNDCP (International Drug Control Program) Interagency Program. Substance Use & Misuse. 1996;**31**:1599-1617

[43] Richmond R, Kehoe L, Heather N, Wodak A. Evaluation of a workplace brief intervention for excessive alcohol consumption: the work screen project. Preventive Medicine. 2000;**30**:51-63

[44] Watson HE, Godfrey C, McFadyen A, McArthur K, Stevenson M. Reducing alcohol-related harm in the workplace: a feasibility study of screening and brief interventions for

hazardous drinkers. Alcohol Education and Research Council. 2009

[45] Hermansson U, Helander A, Brandt L, Huss A, Ronnberg S. Screening and brief intervention for risky alcohol consumption in the workplace: results of a 1 year randomised controlled study. Alcohol and Alcoholism. 2010;**45**:252-257

[46] Zibe-Piegel VP, Boerngen-Lacerda R. How to detect early harmful and hazardous substance use in workplace: A qualitative study. Journal of Alcoholism & Drug Dependence. 2013;**1**(104) [online]. DOI: 10.4172/jaldd.1000104 Accessed: 24 June 2022

[47] Ito C, Yuzuriha T, Noda T, Ojima T, Hiro H, Higuchi S. Brief intervention in the workplace for heavy drinkers: a randomized clinical trial in Japan. Alcohol and Alcoholism. 2015;**50**:157-163

[48] Wilk AI, Jensen NM, Havighurst TC. Meta analysis of randomised control trails addressing brief intervention in heavy alcohol drinker. Journal of Internal Medicine. 1997;**12**:274-283

[49] Ballesteros J, Duffy JC, Querejeta I, Ariño J, González-Pinto A. Efficacy of brief interventions for hazardous drinkers in primary care. Alcoholism, Clinical and Experimental Research. 2004;**28**:608-618

[50] Bertholet N, Daeppen JB, Wietlisbach V, Fleming M, Burnand B. Reduction of alcohol consumption by brief alcohol intervention in primary care. Archives of Internal Medicine. 2005;**165**:986-995

[51] McQueen J, Howe TE, Allan L, Mains D, Hardy V. Brief interventions for heavy alcohol users admitted to general hospital wards. Cochrane Database of Systematic Reviews. 2011;**10**(8):1-56. [online]. DOI: 10.1002/14651858. CD005191.pub3 Accessed: 20 July 2022

[52] Sullivan LE, Tetrault JM, Braithwaite RS, Turner BJ, Fiellin DA. A meta-analysis of the efficacy of non-physician brief interventions for unhealthy alcohol use: implications for the patient-centered medical home. American Journal on Addictions. 2011;**20**:343-356

[53] Cuijpers P, Riper H, Lemmers L. The effects on mortality of brief interventions for problem drinking: a meta-analysis. Addiction. 2004;**99**:839-845

[54] Senft RA, Polen MR, Freeborn DK, Hollis JF. Brief intervention in a primary care setting for hazardous drinkers. American Journal of Preventive Medicine. 1997;**13**:464-470

[55] WHO Brief Intervention Study Group. A randomized cross-national clinical trial of brief interventions with heavy drinkers. American Journal of Public Health. 1996;**86**:948-955

[56] Wutzke SE, Shiell A, Gomel MK, Conigrave KM. Cost effectiveness of brief interventions for reducing alcohol consumption. Social Science & Medicine. 2001;**52**:863-870

[57] Kaner EF, Dickinson HO, Beyer FR, Campbell F, Schlesinger C, Heather N, et al. Effectiveness of brief alcohol interventions in primary care populations. Cochrane Database of Systematic Reviews. 2007;**18**:CD004148

[58] Holloway AS, Watson HE, Arthur AT, Starr G, McFadyen AK, McIntosh J. The effect of brief interventions on alcohol consumption among heavy drinkers in a general hospital setting. Addiction. 2007;**102**:1762-1770

[59] Solberg LI, Maciosek MV, Edwards NM. Primary care intervention

to reduce alcohol misuse. Ranking its health impact and cost effectiveness. American Journal of Preventive Medicine. 2008;**34**:143-152

[60] Henry-Edwards S, Humeniuk S, Ali R, Monteiro M, Poznyak V. Brief Intervention for substance use: A manual for use in primary care. Geneva: World Health Organization; 2003

[61] Lock CA, Kaner E, Heather N, Doughty J, Crawshaw A, McNamee PL. Effectiveness of nurse-led brief alcohol intervention: a cluster randomized controlled trial. Journal of Advanced Nursing 2006; 54: 426-39.

[62] Chang G, McNamara TK, Orav EJ, Koby D, Lavigne A, Ludman B. Brief intervention for prenatal alcohol use: a randomized trial. Obstetrics and Gynecology. 2005;**105**:991-998

[63] Ockene JK, Adams A, Hurley TG, Wheeler EV, Hebert JR. Brief physician and nurse practitioner-delivered counselling for high-risk drinkers: does it work? Archives of Internal Medicine. 1999;**159**:2198-2205

[64] Goodall CA, Ayoub AF, Crawford A, Smith I, Bowman A, Koppel D. Nurse delivered brief interventions for hazardous drinkers with alcohol-related facial trauma: a prospective randomised controlled trial. British Journal of Oral & Maxillofacial Surgery. 2008;**46**:96-101

[65] Pal HR, Yadav D, Mehta S, Mohan IA. Comparison of brief intervention versus simple advice for alcohol use disorders in a North India community-based sample followed for 3 months. Alcohol and Alcoholism. 2007;**42**:328-332

[66] Gryczynski IJ, Mitchell SG, Peterson TR, Gonzales A, Moseley A, Schwartz RP. The relationship between services delivered and substance use outcomes in New Mexico's Screening, Brief Intervention, Referral and Treatment (SBIRT) Initiative. Drug and Alcohol Dependence. 2011;**118**:152-157

[67] Bertha KM, Compton WC, Avula D, Stegbauer T, Stein JB, Clark HW. Screening, brief interventions, referral to treatment (SBIRT) for illicit drug and alcohol use at multiple healthcare sites: comparison at intake and six months. Drug and Alcohol Dependence. 2009;**99**:280-295

[68] Mitchell GS, Gryczynski J, Gonzales A, Moseley A, Peterson T, O'Grady KE, et al. Screening, Brief Intervention, and Referral to Treatment (SBIRT) for Substance Use in a School-based Program: services and outcomes. American Journal on Addictions. 2012;**21**:S5-S13

[69] Bernstein J, Bernstein E, Tassiopoulos K, Heeren T, Levenson S, Hingson R. Brief motivational intervention at a clinic visit reduces cocaine and heroin use. Drug and Alcohol Dependence. 2005;**77**:49-59

[70] Saunders B, Wilkinson C, Phillips M. The impact of a brief motivational intervention with opiate users attending a methadone programme. Addiction. 1995;**90**:415-424

[71] Baer JS, Garrett SB, Beadnell B, Wells EA, Peterson PL. Brief motivational intervention with homeless adolescents: Evaluating effects on substance use and service utilization. Psychology of Addictive Behaviors. 2007;**21**:582-586

[72] Young MM , Stevens A, Galipeau J, Pirie T, Garritty C, Singh K, et al. SBIRT model for reducing the nonmedical use of psychoactive substances: A systematic review. 2014. [online] Available from: http://www.systematicreviews journal.

com/content/3/1/50. [Accessed: 18 July 2022]

[73] Gates P, Copeland J, Swift W, Martin G. Barriers and facilitators to cannabis treatment. Drug and Alcohol Review. 2012;**31**:311-319

[74] Fischer B, Dawe M, McGuire F, Shuper PA, Capler R, Bilsker D, et al. Feasibility and impact of brief interventions for frequent cannabis users in Canada. Journal of Substance Abuse Treatment. 2014;**44**:132-138

[75] Madras BK, Compton WM, Avula D, Stegbauer T, Stein JB, Clark HW. Screening, brief interventions, referral to treatment (SBIRT) for illicit drug and alcohol use at multiple healthcare sites: comparison at intake and 6 months later. Drug and Alcohol Dependence. 2009;**99**:280-295

[76] Martin G, Copeland J. The adolescent cannabis check-up: randomized trial of a brief intervention for young cannabis users. Journal of Substance Abuse Treatment. 2008;**34**:407-414

[77] Stein MD, Hagerty CE, Herman DS, Phipps MG, Anderson BJ. A brief marijuana intervention for non-treatment-seeking young adult women. Journal of Substance Abuse Treatment. 2011;**40**:189-198

[78] Stephens RS, Roffman RA, Curtin L. Comparison of extended versus brief treatments for marijuana use. Journal of Consulting and Clinical Psychology. 2000;**68**:898-908

[79] Walker DD, Stephens R, Roffman R, DeMarce J, Lozano B, Towe S, et al. Randomized controlled trial of motivational enhancement therapy with nontreatment-seeking adolescent cannabis users: a further test of the teen marijuana check-up. Psychology of Addictive Behaviors. 2011;**25**:474-484

[80] Denering LL, Spear SE. Routine use of screening and brief intervention for college students in a university counselingcenter. Journal of Psychoactive Drugs. 2012;**44**:318-324

[81] Spear S, Tilman S, Moss C, Gong-Guy E, Ransom L, Rawson RA. Another way of talking about substance abuse: substance abuse screening and brief intervention in a mental health clinic. Journal of Human Behavior in the Social Environment. 2009;**19**:959-977

[82] Stead LF, Buitrago D, Preciado N, Sanchez G, Hartmann-Boyce J, Lancaster T. Physician advice for smoking cessation. The Cochrane Database of Systematic Reviews. 2013;**5**:CD000165

[83] Humeniuk R, Ali R, Babor T, Souza-Formigoni ML, de Lacerda RB, Ling W, et al. A randomized controlled trial of a brief intervention for illicit drugs linked to the Alcohol, Smoking and Substance Involvement Screening Test (ASSIST) in clients recruited from primary health-care settings in four countries. Addiction. 2012;**107**:957-966

[84] Assanangkornchai S, Balthip Q, Edwards JG. Implementing the alcohol, smoking, substance involvement screening test and linked brief intervention service in primary care in Thailand. Journal of Public Health. 2014;**36**:443-449

[85] Saitz R, Palfai PA, Cheng DM, Daniel P, Bernstein AD, Christine AL, et al. Screening and brief intervention for drug use in primary care. The ASPIRE Randomized Clinical Trial. JAMA. 2014;**312**:502-513

[86] Loretta L, Denering MS, Suzanne ES. Routine use of screening and brief

intervention for college students in a university counseling center. Journal of Psychoactive Drugs. 2012;**44**:318-324

[87] Pengpid S, Peltzer K, Puckpinyo A, Viripiromgool S, Thamma-aphiphol K, Suthisukhon K, et al. Screening and concurrent brief intervention of conjoint hazardous or harmful alcohol and tobacco use in hospital out-patients in Thailand: a randomized controlled trial. Substance Abuse Treatment, Prevention, and Policy. 2015;**10**:22. DOI: 10.1186/s13011-015-0018-1 PMCID: PMC4448213

[88] Lasebikan VO and Ola BA. Community-based screening, brief intervention, and referral for treatment for unhealthy tobacco use: single arm study experience and implementation success in rural and semi-rural settings, South-West Nigeria. Front. Psychiatry. 2016; 7:134. doi: 10.3389/fpsyt.2016.00134 [online] Available from: http//:www.frontiersin.org [Accessed: 17 July 2022]

[89] Joseph J, Das K, Sharma S, Basu D. ASSIST linked alcohol screening and brief intervention in workplace: a feasibility study from a tertiary hospital of North India. Indian Association for Social Psychiatry. 2013;**29**:75-78

[90] Joseph J, Das K, Sharma S, Basu D. ASSIST-linked alcohol screening and brief intervention in Indian workplace setting: result of a 4-month follow up. Indian Association for Social Psychiatry. 2014;**30**:80-86

[91] Prasad S, Basu D, Mattoo SK, Subodh BN. Brief intervention to reduce risky use of psychoactive substances in class c male hospital employees: A randomised controlled trial (indianjpsyc hiatry_660_21;Unpublished DM Thesis)